The International Behavioural and

MENTAL HEALTH IN THE SERVICE OF THE COMMUNITY

TAVISTOCK

The International Behavioural and Social Sciences Library

MENTAL HEALTH
In 8 Volumes

MENTAL HEALTH IN THE SERVICE OF THE COMMUNITY

Volume Three of a Report
of an International and
Interprofessional Study Group
convened by the World
Federation for Mental Health

EDITED BY KENNETH SODDY
AND ROBERT H AHRENFELDT
WITH THE ASSISTANCE OF
MARY C KIDSON

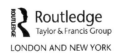 Routledge
Taylor & Francis Group

LONDON AND NEW YORK

First published in 1967 by
Tavistock Publications Limited

Published in 2001 by
Routledge
2 Park Square, Milton Park, Abingdon, Oxfordshire OX14 4RN
711 Third Avenue, New York, NY 10017

First issued in paperback 2014

Routledge is an imprint of the Taylor and Francis Group, an informa business

© 1967 Kenneth Soddy

British Library Cataloguing in Publication Data
A CIP catalogue record for this book
is available from the British Library

Mental Health in the Service of the Community
ISBN 0-415-26456-1
Mental Health: 8 Volumes
ISBN 0-415-26511-8
The International Behavioural and Social Sciences Library
112 Volumes
ISBN 0-415-25670-4

ISBN 13: 978-1-138-86746-8 (pbk)
ISBN 13: 978-0-415-26456-3 (hbk)

Mental Health in the Service of the Community

Volume III of a Report of an International and Interprofessional Study Group convened by the World Federation for Mental Health

Edited by KENNETH SODDY
and ROBERT H. AHRENFELDT
with the assistance of Mary C. Kidson

TAVISTOCK PUBLICATIONS
J. B. LIPPINCOTT COMPANY

First published in 1967
by Tavistock Publications Limited
2 Park Square, Milton Park, Abingdon, Oxon, OX14 4RN
in 11 pt Plantin
by Butler & Tanner Ltd, Frome & London

Distributed in the United States of America and in Canada
by J. B. Lippincott Company, Philadelphia and Montreal

To
JOHN RAWLINGS REES, C.B.E., M.D., F.R.C.P.,
this report in three volumes is affectionately
dedicated by the members of the
International Study Group
on Mental Health Perspectives, 1961

Volume I Mental Health in a Changing World
Volume II Mental Health and Contemporary Thought
Volume III Mental Health in the Service of the Community

Contents

Acknowledgements

Grateful acknowledgement is made to the National Institute of Mental Health, US Public Health Service, for US PHS Research Grant No. M-4998, which made it possible for the International Study Group to meet, for the summary report *Mental Health in International Perspective* to be prepared, and for editorial work on the current report in three volumes to be started; to the Grant Foundation of New York for bearing the cost of the salaries of the members of the Scientific Division of WFMH; to the Council for International Organizations of Medical Sciences for a subvention towards the preparation of resource materials; and to the WFMH US Committee Inc. for a grant towards the completion of the bibliography included in these volumes.

Obituary

ALBERT DEUTSCH died, suddenly and peacefully, in his sleep on Sunday, 18 June 1961, the seventh day in the work programme of the Study Group with which this Report is concerned. He was an experienced science writer and journalist, and perhaps the most distinguished 'communicator' in the field of mental health. His main assignment with the Study Group, in which he also took an active part, was to write the summary report for presentation at the International Congress on Mental Health in Paris, August–September 1961.

For thirty years Albert Deutsch had been completely dedicated to the task of raising the level of understanding in the United States of the problems of mental ill health, and made immense contributions to the promotion of awareness both of the need for change and of means towards its achievement.

Participants

The participants in the International Study Group came from eleven countries and represented fifteen fields of professional work. Their names, and their professional appointments at the time of the Study Group, are listed below:

DR H. C. RÜMKE (*Chairman*)
Professor of Psychiatry, University of Utrecht; Member, Royal Academy of Sciences in the Netherlands

DR ROBERT H. AHRENFELDT
Psychiatrist; Consultant and Research Associate, WFMH; *formerly* Dep. Asst Director of Army Psychiatry, War Office (UK)

THE REV. GEORGE C. ANDERSON
Director, Academy of Religion and Mental Health, New York

DR SIMON BIESHEUVEL
Director, National Institute for Personnel Research, South African Council for Scientific and Industrial Research, Johannesburg

†MR ALBERT DEUTSCH
Editor-in-Chief, *Encyclopaedia of Mental Health*, Washington, D.C.

DR JACK R. EWALT
Professor of Psychiatry, Harvard University Medical School; Superintendent, Massachusetts Mental Health Center; Director, Joint Commission on Mental Illness and Health, USA

DR RICHARD H. FOX
Psychiatrist, Bethlem Royal and Maudsley Hospitals; Hon. Asst Secretary, Research Committee, Mental Health Research Fund, UK; Secretary, Medical Research Council (UK) Sub-committee on Psychopathic Personality

PARTICIPANTS

DR FRANK FREMONT-SMITH
Director, Interdisciplinary Conference Program, American Institute of Biological Sciences; President and Chairman, Governing Board, WFMH US Committee Inc.; Co-Chairman, World Mental Health Year Committee

DR OTTO KLINEBERG
Professor and Chairman, Department of Social Psychology, Columbia University

DR DAVID M. LEVY
Lecturer in Psychiatry, College of Physicians and Surgeons, Columbia University; Consulting Psychiatrist, New York City Dept of Health; Visiting Professor of Psychiatry, Tulane University Medical School, New Orleans

DR TSUNG-YI LIN
Professor of Psychiatry, National Taiwan University Medical College, Taipei, Taiwan

DR STEPHEN A. MACKEITH
Consultant Psychiatrist and Physician Superintendent, Warlingham Park Hospital, Surrey; Adviser in Psychiatry to the County Borough of Croydon, Surrey; Consultant Psychiatrist, Mayday Hospital, Croydon

DR MARGARET MEAD
Visiting Professor of Anthropology, Menninger School of Psychiatry; Associate Curator of Ethnology, American Museum of Natural History; Adjunct Professor of Anthropology, Columbia University; Visiting Professor of Anthropology, School of Psychiatry, College of Medicine, University of Cincinnati

DR BEN S. MORRIS
Professor of Education and Director of the Institute of Education, University of Bristol

DR A. C. PACHECO E SILVA
Professor of Clinical Psychiatry, Faculty of Medicine, University of São Paulo, and School of Medicine of São Paulo; President, WFMH, 1960–61

DR JOHN R. REES
Director, WFMH

DR AASE G. SKARD
Associate Professor, Department of Child Psychology, University of Oslo

DR KENNETH SODDY
Scientific Director, WFMH; Physician and Lecturer in Child Psychiatry, University College Hospital and Medical School, London

DR GEORGE S. STEVENSON
Editor, *Mental Hygiene* (NAMH quarterly); President, WFMH, 1961–62; *formerly* National and International Consultant, NAMH; Medical Director, National Committee for Mental Hygiene, USA

DR ALAN STOLLER
Chief Clinical Officer, Mental Hygiene Authority, State of Victoria, Australia

DR MOTTRAM P. TORRE
Assistant Director, WFMH; Asst Attending Psychiatrist, St Luke's Hospital, New York

DR CLAUDE VEIL
Psychiatre de l'Association Interprofessionnelle des Centres Médicaux du Travail, Paris; Chargé de Conférences Techniques à l'Institut de Psychologie, Paris; Secrétaire du Groupe d'Hygiène Mentale Industrielle (Ligue d'Hygiène Mentale)

WHO Observers:
†DR E. EDUARDO KRAPF
Chief, Mental Health Section, WHO (*died 9 December 1963*)

DR DONALD F. BUCKLE
Regional Officer for Mental Health, WHO, Regional Office for Europe

DR TIGANI EL MAHI
Regional Adviser for Mental Health, WHO, Regional Office for the Eastern Mediterranean

Preface

It is with great pleasure that I have accepted the invitation to write a preface for the Report in three volumes of the International Study Group convened by the World Federation for Mental Health in 1961. For me, as Chairman of the Study Group, the reading of the manuscript has revived many memories of this fascinating meeting and stimulated a great number of thoughts. I believe that the Report is of the greatest importance not only for those of us who had the good fortune to be members of the Study Group, but also for all those who are interested in both the scientific basis and the practice of mental health. In these restless and changing days, with their unending series of unpredictable international tensions, it may reasonably be asked whether it was worth while for a small group of men and women of widely varying individual scientific interests to come together in remote and lovely surroundings merely for the purpose of talking with each other. Although they had prepared working papers for the meeting and a number of references to the literature had been collected, they came without prepared scientific papers, 'official' documents, important statistical findings, films, or other concrete evidence, and also without an agreed conceptual foundation for the meeting. What they did bring with them was their experience of many and various forms of psychiatry, clinical and social psychology, sociology, education, or religion.

Within a prepared framework, which was designed more or less to cover the field of mental health, the Study Group spent its time in extempore discussion ranging over the oldest, the newest, and the most urgent problems of human beings. The conceptual aim of the conference was to provide an open exchange of thoughts, experiences, and views among a group of people of wide and varied experience, and by so doing to make a contribution to the science of man by the integration of the most diverse and highly specialized personal experience. The long-term hope was that the resulting synthesis of experience might make the sciences of man of greater value in the endeavour to improve mental health all over the world.

It is sometimes asked whether it is possible to achieve such ends by merely talking, and whether the not inconsiderable sums of money involved are well spent. Many of those who have been brought up in the natural science disciplines are not in sympathy with this type of programme. Natural scientists today are preoccupied with their attempts to raise the levels of methodological precision, to reach a higher level of objectivity, to clarify their models of thought, and to advance new hypotheses in the search for scientific principles. We can perfectly understand the point of view that the aims of the natural scientist as defined cannot be furthered by group discussion. On the other hand, we hope that many natural scientists are aware of the more intangible factors that appear to be operating in the field of the human mind and of the relationships between people, and that they may be willing to agree that the special conditions obtaining in the field of mental health may require alternative and additional methods of approach.

We would ask the natural science purist who is unable to make any concession to a less pragmatic method of operation not to concern himself overmuch with these volumes. The purist is not likely to find a great deal of value in this Report. He will be distressed by a comparative lack of objectivity, and his scientific self-confidence may lead him into the detection of many errors. Above all, he will be greatly concerned by the lack of scientific proof for much that occupied the International Study Group's time.

Those who took part in the Study Group are fully convinced that such heterogeneous interprofessional and transcultural discussions are of high potential value, provided they are properly prepared and imaginatively planned. It is our conviction that this way of working enables us to arrive at the sources of new thinking. The work in which we are engaged in advancing the scientific knowledge of mental health is still only at its very beginning. The phase in which we are now working may fairly be called 'pre-scientific' – a necessary precursor of more objectively scientific ways of working. In our view, it is premature to narrow our interests to an exclusive specialization and search for objectivity. There is a place for both kinds of work – more concern with objectivity is urgently needed, but at the same time we need to preserve a view of the whole field in order to see more clearly the relative values of the many lines of specialized inquiry.

In this 'pre-scientific' era of mental health work, the primary need is to know how best to relate the many and various findings over the whole range of the field, at a time when much of the practical work that is being carried on is not of a highly specialized order. Major advances in conceptualization are not possible without the cooperation of a multidisciplined team. It has been said with some truth that from multidisciplined to undisciplined thinking is only one step. But, on the other hand, multidisciplinary thinking is the best defence against both the overestimation and the underestimation of the results of single-disciplined work. Only the multidisciplinary approach is likely to lead us to whole and basic truths.

This Report gives a number of perspectives over the whole of human life. Its subject-matter, which ranges widely around the world, will enrich the reader. The great complexity of the material and the diversity of thought may well have a confusing effect, but throughout the Report the connecting factor is the human being – Man as he is today in an ever-changing environment. If the reader is able to keep this connecting thread always in his mind, he will be at the same time surprised at the wide variety of human experience and fascinated by the essential sameness of human beings all over the world.

May I conclude by thanking, in the name of the members of the International Study Group, those who have completed the immense task of compiling these three volumes out of the many

and various records of our discussions: Dr Kenneth Soddy, Dr
Robert H. Ahrenfeldt, and Miss Mary C. Kidson.

Utrecht   H. C. RÜMKE

January 1964

Editors' Introduction

The Report of the International Study Group on Mental Health, 1961, convened by the World Federation for Mental Health, is being published in three volumes.

Volume I – *Mental Health in a Changing World* – describes the background and work methods of the International Study Group, and presents a summary of the Group's recommendations and an account of the major developments and changes in the world-wide mental health field since the publication in 1948 of *Mental Health and World Citizenship*.

Volume II – *Mental Health and Contemporary Thought* – is concerned with the Study Group's discussions on mental health in relation to the contemporary international scene, on the conceptual background to modern mental health work, and on the implications of modern conditions for professional training and public education in this field.

Volume III – *Mental Health in the Service of the Community* – records the Study Group's discussion of current diagnostic, therapeutic, and prophylactic action in the mental health field, and of the more salient aspects of research.

Originally conceived as one volume, the Report was divided into three volumes for the convenience of those readers who are concerned with a limited sector rather than the whole field of mental health. Like other aspects of social concern, the field of mental health action has widened very considerably in the last few decades. The editors believe that those whose main interest is in the promotion of mental health work may find Volume I the most absorbing of the three; those who are concerned with social problems and the light that the modern sciences of Man can throw on them may find Volume II more to their liking;

and those who are engaged in direct therapeutic work, whether individual or community, may prefer Volume III. For the convenience of readers who do not wish to consult the complete set, the bibliography has been included in each of the volumes.

At the present time it is sometimes said that the method of conference discussion is out of fashion and that it can add little or nothing that is new to its subject. Those who set up the International Study Group on Mental Health, 1961, do not share this view; they consider that the conference discussion has fallen out of favour only among those people who have not understood either its full potentialities or the technical requirements for success. It is readily conceded that a conference may be useless, even harmful, if it is not properly prepared for, and if there is no clear idea of the aims; and, indeed, there is far more to a conference than the mere gathering together of people to talk about a subject. In this volume we have discussed some of the difficulties of people currently engaged in mental health work, and have emphasized the necessity for applying insights gained from modern psychology and allied sciences to the work problems involved. This is true of conferences no less than of other aspects of the work. It would not be reasonable, today, to convene a conference on a mental health subject without bringing to it all the insights available from studies of group dynamics.

It is well recognized that intercommunication is achieved most easily in a group that is homogeneous in terms of age, nationality or culture, educational level, and so on; and with the greatest difficulty when the group is markedly heterogeneous. The International Study Group, 1961, was, by design, interprofessional, transnational, and included a wide age-range. Without a considerable degree of heterogeneity, a Study Group on transnational mental health questions would be pointless. The inherent difficulties of heterogeneity were, we believe, successfully offset by the specific experience of the Study Group members. The nucleus around which the Study Group was formed was the Scientific Committee of the Federation, the members of which had been in the habit of meeting regularly over a period of about six years for the purpose of studying and writing reports on emerging mental health topics. This group was highly practised in intercommunication; and those members of the International Study Group who were not on the Scientific Committee, though not so closely organized at the outset, also brought with them a wealth of experience of communication across cultural and professional frontiers, and in every case were well known professionally to one or more members of the Scientific Committee.

Thus the Study Group, though apparently heterogeneous, and though coming from many different professions and nations, had in fact achieved a degree of homogeneity of interest in the mental health field before it started its work. The effect of this was quickly visible in the highly integrated work that the Study Group was able to accomplish within a period of two weeks.

Editors of reports are faced with the difficult choice of how far to reproduce verbatim records of discussions and how far to attempt to make a distillate. In the present instance we have tried to achieve a compromise between the extremes. Tape recordings were made of the entire discussions and, in addition, the members themselves had provided a number of working papers and annotations for the editors to draw upon. The main task of the editors has been to arrange the discussions in what appeared to them to be the most logical order, and then to write a considered commentary on the material, illustrating it where appropriate with extracts from the tape recordings and working papers.

The members of the Study Group have voluntarily accepted a group responsibility for what is written in these three volumes. Every member of the Group has had an opportunity to read and comment on the draft and, as far as possible, all the comments received have been acted upon by the editors. That these three volumes represent the agreed Report of the twenty-four members of the Study Group is true in spirit rather than in detail. It is not conceivable that every member agrees with every word that has been written, and in some instances the areas of individual disagreement may be quite wide. Wherever a known area of disagreement or open controversy has been touched upon in the text the editors have attempted to make this clear to the reader.

The editors have been at pains to ensure that the extensive bibliography is accurate and complete up to the summer of 1962. A few books published since that time have been brought to our notice and we have included these under the heading 'Supplementary Titles' but we lacked the facilities to ensure that the list of recent additions is complete.

The editors wish to record their very deep indebtedness to all the members of the Study Group, who have responded so willingly and generously to all requests made for working papers and for criticism and comments on the draft of this Report. A great deal of work has been put into these volumes by a large number of people. We are, of course, most particularly indebted to our Chairman, Professor Dr H. C. Rümke, for his guiding hand throughout the operation and for his highly valued contributions to the compilation of the Report.

We should like to add our own personal note of gratitude to our Editorial Assistant, Miss Mary Kidson, for her immense help throughout, and especially in organizing the very complex material in the later stages of report writing. To her name we would add the names of Miss Elizabeth Barnes, for providing a framework for the first draft of the Report, and Mr Peter Robinson, for his invaluable assistance with the bibliography.

We have found the compilation of this Report a most stimulating and extending experience, and we hope that it will give the reader some notion of the rich field of work to be found in mental health all over the world today.

London   KENNETH SODDY
January 1964   ROBERT H. AHRENFELDT

Note to Volume III

This volume completes the report in three volumes of the wfmh International Study Group of 1961. As stated in the Editors' Introduction, the first volume is devoted mainly to a description of the major trends in the field of mental health since 1948, and subsequent to the report of the International Preparatory Commission of the Third International Congress on Mental Health, entitled *Mental Health and World Citizenship*. During the years under review the focus of attention in mental health work has moved from the immediate postwar preoccupation with reparation for the damage to human relationships suffered during the war to a more forward-looking perspective on current social and individual problems.

In Volume II the editors have computed an interpretive record of the Study Group's discussions about modern mental health insights and their application to the world scene. They have discussed the evolution of the concept of mental health itself and the various kinds of professional training and public education in these matters required today. To quote from the Note to Volume II, there has been a 'modest but very serious attempt to apply the knowledge and skill gained in professional work on mental health problems to the problems of living in a world suddenly made small by the enormous improvement in communications and more and more crowded by the steep rise in world population'.

In Volume III the editors have brought together the International Study Group's many discussions about multiprofessional action in the field of mental health for the individual and in the community, in diagnosis, therapy, prophylaxis, and research. Mental health work is rapidly developing in many parts of the world, and involving the members of more and more professional disciplines employed in perhaps a hundred or more independent administrations. In the circumstances it follows that the information available to the International Study Group has been neither exhaustive nor highly accurate. The notorious difficulties of information collection have greatly increased our already heavy debt of gratitude to all those who have supplied us with material. Thanks are due to the various members of the Study Group for their individual contributions; in addition, we are heavily indebted to the late Dr E. E. Krapf and Mrs Joy Moser of the Mental Health Section of WHO in Geneva for the fact-finding work that they undertook on our behalf; to Dr Donald Buckle of WHO European Region; to Bio-Sciences Information Exchange in Washington; to the United States Public Health Service; and to many other sources of information.

However incomplete, the information made available to the International Study Group shows ample evidence of the vigorous expansion of mental health action in a large number of countries and in many directions. New treatment methods in conjunction with increasingly liberal attitudes to the problem of the mentally ill are contributing to major revolutions in diagnostic, therapeutic, rehabilitatory, and custodial practices.

Inevitably, these new potentialities and opportunities for mental health action are accompanied by new responsibilities and problems. Perhaps the paramount issue is that of the integration of psychiatric treatment more fully into the normal practices and provisions of society. If cases of mental illness are to receive the early recognition that modern treatment methods deserve and demand, it is essential that the sufferer should no longer be regarded as an individual apart, as he still is in many instances. If, on the other hand, society comes to expect the early return home of the hospitalized patient but demands as a condition the total masking of symptoms and signs by pharmacological methods, more harm than good may be done.

Another current problem area concerns the introduction of modern psychiatric techniques to newly developing countries where resources of professionally trained personnel are limited or in many cases virtually non-existent. The principles governing the application of experience gained in one set of circumstances to other and rapidly changing conditions are little understood and their further elucidation is a modern imperative.

The least adequate section of this volume is that devoted to research. Even if full allowance is made for the admitted incompleteness of our information, it can hardly be disputed that the interdisciplinary research that is being undertaken in the mental health field is inadequate both in quantity and in quality to sustain the healthy and rapid expansion of mental health action. Interdisciplinary research is necessarily concerned with areas on the borderline of interest of each profession involved; it demands an originality of conceptualization that is unlikely to arise spontaneously from nothing, but needs to be fostered and developed as experience grows. There is no more pressing task in the mental health field today than that of raising the level of research work.

Whatever the shortcomings, nevertheless, the growth of mental health work in the last two decades has been remarkable all over the world, and it is the hope of the editors and of all the members of the International Study Group that the account given in these pages may prove useful in preparing for still further advances.

PART ONE

Diagnostic, Therapeutic, and Prophylactic Action

I
Governmental Action

TRENDS IN CLINICAL AND
COMMUNITY MENTAL HEALTH SERVICE PLANNING
Since the end of World War II, a large number of studies have
been attempted in many parts of the world of current problems,
existing services, and possible future requirements in the field
of mental health. The transnational material on which future
planning can be based is necessarily heterogeneous, comprising
reports on various cultures, and on different conditions and
stages of social and economic development. But even the most
cursory glance at a selection of material from all over the world
reveals an almost universal preoccupation with and awareness of
a shortage of mental hospital beds, the inadequacy of clinical
facilities for inpatients and outpatients, and a great deficiency as
regards the required numbers of suitably trained professional
personnel. This concern appears to be shared not only by
countries of Western Europe and North America, but also by
countries in other parts of the world where psychiatric work is of
more recent origin.

Anything more than a superficial study of the facts reveals a
serious lack of knowledge, almost everywhere, as to specific
requirements of mental health services in particular cultures,
populations, and localities (urban and rural). In a number of
countries, notably the United Kingdom (103) and the United
States (160, 384), certain standards have been established with
regard to the numbers of psychiatric hospital beds and personnel
required in proportion to the population; and comparable standards have, in general, been found to be applicable to other
countries in Western Europe. However, it is increasingly realized
that such standards can be laid down only in relation to current

3

therapeutic measures and, more particularly, to current public attitudes to psychiatric treatment.

The evidence of need has appeared sufficiently clear for a WHO Expert Committee on Mental Health (195) to recommend, tentatively, the minimal number of essential psychiatric beds 'which any country, regardless of its level of economic development, should aim to provide' for the segregation and treatment of cases requiring hospitalization. The committee's recommendation was made after considering the experience of psychiatrists working in various parts of Asia and tropical Africa.

Even in the countries where these matters have been most thoroughly investigated, it is still possible only to guess at the incidence and prevalence of mental disorders in the community as a whole. In general, large-scale statistics refer only to patients who have attended hospitals or outpatient clinics. They do not enable other than crude judgements to be made about real prevalence, or about basic aetiology, social environment, or other factors. While data remain limited, planning is bound to continue to be largely empirical.

This applies with even greater force to countries where psychiatric services are less developed. There, the whole field of mental health is open to question and innovation in respect of types of hospital requirement, and number and types of personnel. The dangers of making generalizations about the needs of whole geographical areas, or even the whole world, are well recognized. Krapf and Moser (5) have emphasized the need, when planning psychiatric services, to have a central mental health agency, directed by a psychiatrist, to plan, stimulate, and foster the overall mental health programme so that it is integrated with the more local mental health programmes of each area. Several authors stress the value, in addition to central planning, of the regionalization of services, so as to meet more adequately the particular requirements of different areas (McKerracher, 146; Le Guillant et al., 209; Sivadon and Duchêne, 383). In his critical review of the literature prepared for the WFMH International Study Group, Ahrenfeldt has underlined the need for a wider range of interdisciplinary planning, to include cultural anthropologists, social psychologists, statisticians, social economists, and so on (see also Stoller, 83). The report of the meeting of specialists on mental health at Bukavu in 1958 (88) is an illustration of 'central' mental health planning for underdeveloped countries.

There have been some highly significant advances in planning in a number of European and North American countries in the last two decades, in the general directions of expansion of community services, promotion of mental health and prevention of ill health, early detection and treatment of mental illness, and rehabilitation. These have encouraged research and training of specialized personnel; and have led to the extension of consultation, emergency, and advisory services; of domiciliary services, outpatient services, day and night hospitals, half-way houses, hostels, clubs, and sheltered workshops.

It is being increasingly recognized that mental health services can be made more effective in prevention and therapy if they are less isolated from other community services. For example, many problems that are brought to their attention might be more effectively dealt with by other agencies, such as general medical and public health services, education, and the social services; or by religious guidance, legal counselling, or correctional agencies. Every agency that deals with people in need or in trouble is concerned with mental health work, and it is emphasized that the psychiatric services can learn from these agencies as well as give them help.

An inquiry into mental health resources and planned priorities was carried out in thirty-three countries by WHO in 1960 (Krapf and Moser (5)). Although the data from this investigation are necessarily incomplete and sometimes subjective, they are of considerable interest, and frequent references will be made to this material in the course of this volume. As a foretaste, it may be noted that, in spite of the importance given by WHO (among other authorities) to the establishment of central mental health direction, only twenty of the countries that cooperated in the inquiry had any central direction, and it can be further assumed that those countries that did not cooperate are unlikely to have set up a central administrative structure for their mental health services. On the whole, where there is central planning, the tendency is to integrate a mental health division fully into the public health services of the country, and in several countries this type of integration is reflected at the local level in the structure of the hospital services.

In a number of countries considerable interest is being shown in the organization of mental health services on a regional basis, as a means of reaching a larger proportion of the population. Current Swedish thinking envisages what is referred to as 'a plan for the "infiltration of society" with mental health attitudes in many activities'. Briefly, it is based on the provision of many small psychiatric hospitals, built in close contact with general hospitals and offering extensive extramural services. In Canada, the incorporation of regional psychiatric hospitals as part of general hospital complexes is being freely advocated. This has also been the case in some of the hospital regions of the United Kingdom, especially where (as is sometimes happening) existing old-fashioned buildings no longer required for their original purpose (e.g. tuberculosis and infectious fever hospitals) are being converted for use as psychiatric hospitals within general hospital complexes. Many countries are seeking to involve the general practitioner to a greater degree, and other measures are being adopted with a view to promoting continuity of care and treatment at all stages of rehabilitation and reintegration into society.

Many other examples of new trends in planning might be given, but a word of warning is necessary about the application of experience in one country to the problems of another. Thus, reporting on a study tour of services in the Soviet Union, Wortis (87) remarked of one institution: 'Treatment wards sometimes seemed crowded, homey and unorganized. Hospital tempo was slow, with manpower lavish and wasted.' However, in a further comment on the same institution, the author wrote: 'The hospital atmosphere always reflected kindness, humanity

6

and an orientation to the needs of patients. The patients – children and adults alike – looked secure in the hospital setting and I did not see any of the forlorn neglected creatures so often found in our own public hospitals.' That the author should at the same time observe that the Russian hospital was 'homey' and complain that hospital patients in the United States may appear forlorn and neglected illustrates one of the pitfalls in the making of cross-cultural comparisons. For, if the American concept of a hospital were that of a homey place, it would be more than likely that American hospitals would reflect this concept generally in their atmosphere. But they do not, and so, presumably, 'homeyness' is not part of the American image of hospital treatment, aims, and objectives. Before making intercultural comparisons, the observer should bear in mind in each case the image of the hospital in the community and the local conventions about staffing, manpower, and personnel roles.

With the above warning in mind, it will be useful to refer briefly to current mental health planning trends in two countries in which considerable developments have occurred over the last two decades: the United States and the United Kingdom.

SOME MENTAL HEALTH PLANNING TRENDS
IN THE UNITED STATES

Planning for health in the United States shows a remarkable diversity, which is not surprising in view of the prevailing theory of government of that country. In a working paper, Ewalt wrote:

'The reason for this multiple responsibility is the belief that matters of health (and education also) are of local concern, and the larger government agencies (State and Federal) assume responsibility only when there is clear demonstration of inadequacy at the private agency and local government levels, plus requests for aid from the particular local community. . . . The state government's powers are limited to general supervision of the quality of the hospitals and the health practitioners through licensing laws. The federal government can intrude only when food, materials, or livestock that cross national or state boundaries constitute some health hazards.'

This diversity is even more marked in the case of mental health than in general health programmes, since in most states mental health is not under a health authority, and the pattern of its organization varies.

It is important to understand this theoretical governmental position before attempting to assimilate lessons from recent American experience. Public resistance to state and federal government planning in health matters in the United States is perhaps balanced by the sense of concern for the public welfare of private citizens, acting singly and in organized groups. Thus, following the United States Mental Health Study Act of 1955, citizen involvement became organized in the Joint Commission on Mental Illness and Health, which was composed of thirty-six large citizens' organizations representing professional, lay, and religious organizations, and also governmental agencies. The report of the Joint Commission (389) indicates both the magnitude of the problem to be faced and the solutions proposed. In his working paper, Ewalt, who was Director of the United States Joint Commission on Mental Illness and Health, wrote:

'We made on site studies of fifteen representative counties selected as typical for certain aspects of US life. As suspected, where lacking in formal mental health services, the communities sought to improvise with existing resources. In general the services offered were inadequate. The family physicians, the clergy, the health department nurses and welfare department social workers tried to cope with the problems presented. In almost all communities the need for expert help was expressed, but only a small proportion had any specific plan for organizing such services.

'Improvement in skills for handling mental health problems by added training for public health nurses, family physicians, social workers, and school counselors will increase the effectiveness of these informal community programs. As psychiatrists become available to do consultation and some direct service with these agencies, they will become an even more important resource for care of the mentally ill.

'In our survey, persons worried or troubled sought help from the clergy more often than any other professional group. A study of the function of the church in mental health reveals that the amount of time spent in counseling, and the training for the work, varies greatly among the individual clergymen. There was a general belief that more preparation for counseling would tend to increase their efficiency. Some believed that too much counseling diluted their parish work for which they were better prepared.

'In some communities the public schools have endeavoured to aid in mental health promotion by training teachers and guidance counselors in techniques believed to foster mental health. Some have used a special organization of subject matter to further this process.'

Although such public attitudes to federal and state action in the mental health field have created problems which are still far from negligible today, remarkable progress has been made since the end of World War II. The first federal landmark was the passage of the National Mental Health Act of 1946, which launched what is now known as the National Mental Health Program, administered by the National Institute of Mental Health, formally founded in April 1949. Another powerful influence upon public opinion was the extensive and enlightened programme in the field of mental illness conducted by the Veterans' Administration.

The National Institute of Mental Health (NIMH) is one of thirteen Divisions (1963) of the National Institutes of Health, grouped around a Clinical Centre fully equipped with laboratories and research facilities, and actively in collaboration with offices for research, programme planning, and training.

The NIMH is engaged on a five-point programme:

1. *Research* into all aspects of mental illness, including somatic,

psychological, and social factors which affect human behaviour; and evaluation of treatment, prevention, and rehabilitation. The Institute itself undertakes research, and it also gives research grants to independent investigators in university and other research centres, to public and private mental health agencies, and to educational and professional organizations for community-based studies.

2. *Training*: there is an acute shortage of qualified mental health personnel in all areas of professional activity, including clinical services, teaching, research, consultation, and administration. The NIMH training programme is directed towards increasing the number of specialists and improving the quality of training in the mental health field generally; extending the mental health content in the curricula of medical schools, graduate schools of public health, and collegiate schools of nursing; and improving the mental health training of other cooperating professions.

The NIMH supports training through teaching grants to universities and other training centres, provision of stipends to graduate students, and grants to promising young scientists for research training and to young specialists in various disciplines for training in community work. More recent activities include the development of interdisciplinary training – of biologists and social scientists, for example – and of training in psychiatry for general practitioners and general physicians; and support is being given on a pilot basis for appropriate training programmes for members of other professions – ministers, lawyers, and educators.

3. *Community services*: the goal is effective programmes for promoting mental health, preventing mental disease, and rehabilitating the mentally ill. Emphasis is placed on such problems as ageing, alcoholism, delinquency, drug addiction, and mental retardation, and on early dissemination of knowledge about research findings.

The main way in which the NIMH can help state administrations is through the procedure laid down by the National Mental

Health Act, whereby states must match each federal dollar given from grants-in-aid with one dollar from their own funds. Each state appoints one of its agencies as the Mental Health Authority responsible for receiving and administering federal grant-in-aid funds, and the state agency staff are responsible for planning community mental health programmes. These include the mental health education of the public, consultation services for professional groups and social agencies generally, rehabilitation of former mental patients, expansion of clinical facilities, and acceleration of activities for the prevention and treatment of alcoholism, drug addiction, and other special mental health problems. Major emphasis has been placed on establishing services at the local community level. A number of states have played a leading part in instituting mental health programmes, notably the state of New York (66, 101).

The Health Amendment Act of 1956 has stimulated additional means of expanding programmes, particularly from the standpoint of treatment and rehabilitation. Grants have been made to government and private state and local agencies, institutions, hospitals, and so on, to encourage and improve methods of case recognition, care, treatment, and rehabilitation.

In addition to grants, the NIMH provides professional technical assistance to states, including help with experimental programmes and pilot schemes, and consultation services to plan and evaluate the programmes. At the request of the state governor the Institute conducts surveys of problems.

The research grant programme of the NIMH operates at a state and community level as well as at the federal level, and the same applies to the training programme of personnel.

4. *Programme development*: the Institute carries on continuous programme development activities over the whole field of mental health. The major areas receiving consideration include rehabilitation, drug addiction, problems of ageing, juvenile delinquency, mental retardation, alcoholism, child-rearing practices and beliefs, student mental health, industrial mental health, accident

prevention, and the impact of urban and suburban life on mental health.

5. *Public education*: the NIMH is engaged in planning and carrying out a broad programme of education utilizing all the communication media. Among the activities is the preparation of pamphlets, study kits, leaflets, brochures, reference lists, film guides, exhibits, and set displays for professional and lay audiences on mental health subjects. There is a programme of dissemination of information about new research findings and effective mental health programme procedures. Assistance and consultation are provided on request to science writers, magazine editors, radio and television producers, and others who are preparing material on mental health and related subjects for publication.

Since the passage of the Mental Health Act the number of outpatients' clinics in this field in the United States has increased threefold; in contrast, since 1955 the previously increasing trend in the number of patients resident in public mental hospitals has been reversed and is now declining at an average rate of about 1·1 per cent per annum. This is in line with similar trends in other countries (see the next section), and is attributable to recent changes in therapeutic approach.

MENTAL HEALTH PLANNING IN THE UNITED KINGDOM
Health planning in the United Kingdom in recent years has followed a different course from that pursued in the United States. Planning has become the concern of the whole community, the government taking the lead, but involving responsible community participation at all levels, nationally and regionally.

These developments have been both a cause and an effect of the so-called welfare state legislation, starting in the first decade of the twentieth century with the provision of limited health insurance schemes, and culminating, at the close of World War II, in compulsory national insurance which forms the basis of a national health service, paid for partly by insurance contributions and partly out of general taxation.

More specific central planning for mental health services has increased steadily over the last three decades, starting with a wartime survey (103), and given impetus by, *inter alia*, the National Health Service Act, 1946, and the Mental Health Act, 1959. Broadly speaking, the effect of these two Acts in the mental health field has been, first, to make the mental health service an integral part of the general medical services of the community; and, second, to define the responsibilities and duties of hospital and local health authorities in the provision of comprehensive mental health services, with a range extending from prophylaxis prevention, and the promotion of community mental health in a positive sense, on the one hand, to recognition, diagnostic treatment, rehabilitation, and reintegration into the community, on the other.

Many of the developments in the mental health services consequent upon the legislative activity of the post-war period are still in progress, and many others have yet to be elaborated, initiated, and tested by practical experience.

Kathleen Jones (376), in her most interesting and scholarly account of mental health and social policy in England from 1845–1959, has well summarized the situation as follows:

'It is not easy to separate the inevitable teething troubles of a new service from permanent and intractable problems, or ephemeral fashions in thought and practice from long-term progress. Future assessment of these eleven complex years may find trends where at present there is only confusion and contradiction, points of emphasis which a contemporary survey overlooks. . . . The great change since 1949 has been the entry of statutory authorities into the field of community work, and the consequent change in the role of voluntary organizations. Local authority Mental Health Departments have begun to shoulder the burden of community care. Mental hospitals have taken up the theme of "community" in two ways – by the development of a dynamic within the hospital which enables it to approximate more closely to the society from which its patients are drawn, and by the development of extramural psychiatric services which bridge the gap

13

between total hospitalization and local authority care. . . .
Since 1948, local authority care, day and night hospitals,
sheltered workshops and other experimental forms of care
have done much to break down the old distinction between
being totally well (at home) and totally sick (in hospital).
We have begun to provide a flexible range of services to meet
the varying needs of individuals.'

Many people in the United Kingdom consider the greatest
obstacle to the development of a full range of community services to be the artificial administrative division between general
practitioner, hospital, and public health services, respectively,
which was introduced by the National Health Service Act. It may
be that, as Jones (376) observes, 'this was the price which had
to be paid for an integrated health service', but the structure
adopted has posed a serious problem which it is essential to solve:
how to ensure that the public is served in a coordinated way. The
generally unsatisfactory position, in so far as it affects the otherwise promising developments in the British mental health services, has been clearly stated by Hargreaves (393):

'On discharge from hospital, the patient's after-care, resettlement, and rehabilitation was made a function of the local
authority by the same Act which removed from it the administration of the mental hospitals. This function was not
made an obligation of the local authority but was merely the
subject of permissive powers. Small wonder that this aspect
of the care of the psychiatric patient, which unlike the hospital
service forms a charge on the rates, should have been neglected
by many authorities. Even had it not been, and even had it been
extensively developed, the problem would remain. How can
continuity of care be provided for the psychiatric patient with
such a division of responsibilities between authorities whose
boundaries bear no relationship to each other? . . . . By virtue
of the characteristics of psychiatric disorders and the extent to
which they manifest themselves in the social sphere as difficulties in living, continuity of care seems essential throughout

the process of treatment, rehabilitation, and resettlement. During this process the patient may be at times an out-patient, at times an in-patient. He will need the help of his family doctor, the psychiatrist, the social worker, the rehabilitation centre, the training centre, at different times. Psychiatry must aim to knit together each of these at present disparate elements in a patient's treatment to provide continuity of treatment, supervision, care, and aid. The obstacles are great. The functional organization of services often runs counter to the varying needs of a patient at different times.'[1]

Notwithstanding these and other difficulties, there is general agreement that the mental health services in Britain are in a healthy state of rapid development, though the situation is complicated by the practical issue of reconciling strict legal interests with psychiatric needs in those cases where admission to hospital involves compulsion. The Acts of Parliament which govern these services in the United Kingdom attempt to resolve this dilemma, but it does not always prove easy in practice. In this regard, the Mental Health Act of 1959, though in some ways hardly more than a tidying-up of legal procedures in respect of mental hospital patients, has proved a considerable help by giving unequivocal recognition to psychiatry as an integral part of medicine, and to the mental health services as part of the health services generally. It is now fully established that treatment for mental disorder and care and training for mental deficiency are available without formality in the same way as treatment for any other illness or condition needing medical care.

There have been some striking trends in the United Kingdom in the last decade in relation to easier admission and discharge from mental hospitals, reduction of numbers of patients in hospital, vastly increased turnover of patients, and proliferation of measures for home care. Current trends in the development of the services include the replacement of older, large hospitals by small units, often in connexion with a general hospital; reduction of the

[1] Cf. the report of a Medical Working Party on a plan for the co-ordinated development of the mental health services of Edinburgh (100).

barriers between the mental patient and the community; better outpatient facilities, day and night hospitals, aftercare and community services; and more vigorous rehabilitation and reintegration measures.

OTHER COUNTRIES WITH HIGHLY DEVELOPED PSYCHIATRIC SERVICES

The Study Group was of the view that in countries where there are more developed psychiatric services, and where the general evolutionary trends show a homogeneity of principle and aim in mental health policy and planning, there is considerable advantage to be derived from making use of the many differences of opinion that exist in respect of clinical methods and their specific details. It is highly desirable to maintain flexibility in the approach to administrative and clinical problems, and to avoid stereotyped and standardized attitudes which can result in a general sterility of development.

Weaknesses remain, moreover, in the countries that are more highly organized and also, in varying degree, in those that are less developed or grossly underdeveloped in this field: a shortage of mental hospital accommodation, insufficient and frequently inadequate clinical facilities for inpatients and outpatients, severely limited community services, and a very great deficiency of suitably trained personnel.

What is even more basic, there is also a serious and widespread lack of knowledge as to what is required, in very different and highly specific cultural and social conditions, in order to provide adequate and locally appropriate psychiatric services.

INTERGOVERNMENTAL REGIONAL ACTION

There is much to be learnt from a review of the activity in the field of mental health of the WHO Regional Office for Europe. This was the first of the WHO Regional Offices to inaugurate a mental health programme.

In the Annual Report, 1959–60, of the Director of the WHO Regional Office for Europe, Buckle has reviewed ten years of mental health programmes. He warns that exact evaluation of programmes is not possible, even if a quantifiable measure of change in a mental health index could be adduced as evidence of the role of any particular agency in bringing about that change. He regards it as an essential function of WHO to spread knowledge through direct consultation, seminars, fellowships, and so on, and, as a matter of principle, to use in these activities not only knowledge that follows from strict research, but knowledge that derives from informed speculation and the construction of hypotheses as well. Buckle writes:

'In ten years the European Office of WHO organized nineteen meetings in the mental health field and participated in the organization of twenty-seven others (one by WFMH; twenty-one by UN; three by UNESCO). Over 700 different participants attended the WHO-sponsored meetings and more than 100 different lecturers have been engaged. The fields of discussion have ranged from nursing to alcoholism, from child guidance to gerontology, from mental hospital practice to public health work, from techniques of treatment to techniques of prevention. From this large number of persons come many reports of changing points of view, of changing practices, of the spreading of new ideas, of the initiation of national training courses, and demands for more fellowships.'

Sometimes WHO's action has been in response to a request from a particular country, or to requests for fellowships for study of particular problems. One of the most useful results of the WHO fellowships programme has been the publication of numerous articles in professional European journals. Buckle also comments on the

'marked increase in the recognition that public health programmes of all kinds are required to take account of factors of mental health and mental illness; general hospitals, child health centres and polyclinics now, as a rule, incorporate psychiatric services in their plans. Nowhere has this appreciation of the mental health element in public health been more evident than in the work of WHO itself. European meetings concerned with rehabilitation, gerontology, cardiac diseases, hospital services, child health, public health nursing, health education, occupational health and refugees – to name only the most prominent – have included mental health experts as consultants and lecturers; the integration of mental health principles with all facets of health work has been exemplified in Regional meetings and can also be demonstrated in national programmes.

'Work in the field of child mental health has been a special feature of the European Office's programmes. The direct products of our activities include two published books (283, 430) and innumerable articles; research supported in the first instance by WHO has led to substantial grants from outside sources for its continuance; child guidance clinics supported in part by WHO have become national institutions; a professional society has been formed as a result of a training course administered by WHO (the Spanish–Portuguese Society for Psycho-analysis); plans for setting up comprehensive child mental health services have been developed in consultation with this Office and will continue to receive WHO consultant advice; the seminars organized on subnormal children have created interest even beyond Europe. It is probably in child mental health that immediate results have been most marked and most pervasive; during the ten years of our work our leadership role has been vindicated by the upsurge of national and international activity in child psychiatry, through the setting up of international professional organizations and through extensions and diversifications of national services '

Another aspect of the work of WHO's European Office has been the involvement of mental health specialists in programmes on the following subjects:

Organization and practice of public health, including rural public health
The hospital in the community

Occupational health services in industrial units
The health of seafarers
School health services
The child in hospital
Prevention of accidents to children
Care of the aged
The epidemiological study of circulatory disease
Rehabilitation of children and adults
Nutrition
Basic and post-basic training of nurses, general and special
Health education of the public.

There has been growing cooperation of public health doctors, nurses, and general practitioners with mental health workers in the day-to-day work of prevention, detection, and treatment of mental illness, and in the spreading of information about modern trends in treatment of the mentally ill; also, a wider range of professional people are cooperating, from such varied fields of work as juvenile delinquency and antisocial behaviour, and the mental health of refugees.

In the very different conditions obtaining in the Eastern Mediterranean Region of WHO, where a mental health adviser has more recently been appointed, the approach has been necessarily somewhat different; and it appears to be a great strength of the present organization of WHO work that the regions are autonomous in many respects, particularly in regard to technical policy. One interesting innovation has been the appointment of a highly qualified European-trained psychiatrist as an adviser, in the first place, to a single country, in the hope that it may be possible to transfer him, after about two years, to another country within the same cultural group, and from thence perhaps elsewhere. In this way it may be feasible to set up a more highly specialized advisory service than would have been possible by operating solely at a regional level. In the Eastern Mediterranean Region the question of cooperation with voluntary agencies is very difficult, because of the lack of resources of the latter. Work in the Region is also handicapped by a relative lack of reliable statistical information and by a dearth of professionally skilled workers.

Underlying all these varied activities is the principle that the duty of WHO lies primarily in the promotion of knowledge, with the objective that the benefits of advances in one country may be made available to others. Only the most expert handling on the part of the Secretariat can further these aims, and the Study Group wished to draw attention to the distinguished work of the various specialized staff members of WHO in this respect. The more recent appointment of a mental health officer to the Regional Office for the Americas was warmly welcomed by the Study Group.

Although the World Federation for Mental Health, no less than the World Health Organization, is deeply committed to the principle of transmission of knowledge and skills across cultural and national frontiers, it cannot be claimed that this aspect of the work of the international agencies, both governmental and non-governmental, has progressed much beyond its infancy. The Study Group was acutely conscious of the many warnings that have been given of the danger of making 'comprehensive' assessments and generalizations; and of the rashness of assuming, in the absence of adequate knowledge, that 'universally' applicable plans for the development of mental health services can suit different cultures, still less whole geographical regions or, indeed, the whole world. There is general agreement that, in each instance, psychiatrists, administrators, and public health authorities need to be guided by the expert knowledge, based on comparative research, of cultural anthropologists and social psychologists; and they need, too, the assistance of statisticians, social economists, and so on.

Krapf (3) observes that, while the scope of international mental health activities is most encouraging,

'it would be a serious mistake if the case for an international approach were overstated. Obviously, it is often possible to establish comparisons between the mental health problems in different areas. Certainly it is frequently possible to use in one part of the world solutions which have proved to be valuable in others. But precisely the international experience of the last ten years has shown very clearly that there are limits to the possibility of comparing situations and of copying solutions . . . that being mentally healthy may have a very different meaning (for people living in different cultural environments). There is, indeed, ample evidence to show that the thoughtless modification of social structures and indiscriminate introduction of new cultural values into a society are capable of causing serious damage to the mental health of its members. This risk exists, of course, also in respect of mental health recommendations which are not in accordance with the value systems of the society in question. The simple transfer of solutions from one area to another is therefore often strongly contra-indicated.'

The hazards of adopting in one country the organization and programmes of another are well recognized, not only because of differing cultural patterns but also because there are, as yet, too few places where mental health activities have been undertaken over a long enough period of time to permit conclusions to be drawn about the consistency of changes of emphasis and direction, or about the effectiveness of courses of action.

Reference has been made to the report of the meeting of specialists on mental health at Bukavu in 1958 (88); it illustrates many of the problems that need to be faced and solved in planning mental health services for countries which are underdeveloped in these respects and which differ very greatly in their cultures and economy. Stoller (83) has also described some of the difficulties and basic principles involved.

Ten years earlier, the International Preparatory Commission of 1948 (12) had recognized in its report the need for flexibility and for attention to local cultural requirements when planning for mental health services in countries without psychiatric facilities. Its view has been well borne out in the years that have followed, when the need for caution in approaching the numerous problems involved has been underlined with the emergence of increasing numbers of new nations. The 1961 Study Group was convinced of the danger of any attempt to establish a mental health service in all its complexity before an adequate assessment of the specific cultural and local requirements had been made.

The statements of the 1948 International Preparatory Commission in this connexion, though mainly relevant today, require certain modifications based on more recent experience. It is now realized, for example, that countries with highly developed mental health services tend to retain, among the practices that have become institutionalized, a number that have originated at earlier stages of advancing knowledge and have, more currently, been seen to be undesirable – such as very large mental hospitals, prolonged custodial care, single methods of therapy applied without reference to individual differences, and so on. Modern methods of social analysis should facilitate the recognition of such harmful institutionalized practices for what they really are, and should prevent their senseless repetition in other parts of the world.

In these days of greatly improved international communications there is an increasing danger of a too rapid and uncritical acceptance by emerging nations of procedures that are new to them. In many cases such procedures may have represented no more than a temporary fashion in the country of their origin, where they may have been insufficiently tested, and their suitability for introduction into very different cultures and situations not evaluated in any way. Among a number of such instances cited by members of the Study Group were: the acquisition of expensive and complex apparatus (e.g. a multichannel electro-encephalograph) without the technical personnel necessary for its effective use; the copying of types of hospital architecture inappropriate to local needs and conditions; and the introduction into one country of psychological tests developed in another, without modification or revalidation.

Turning from the more abstract and scientific sphere to consider the field of practical action for mental health, the Study Group was of the opinion that nowhere has the maximum use been made by governmental agencies of voluntary agencies in the mental health field. It was pointed out that the harnessing of local voluntary effort for the good of the community is of particular importance in the sphere of interpersonal relations.

The work of intergovernmental agencies in mental health necessarily overlaps to some extent the work of voluntary agencies. The latter will be discussed more extensively in the next section, but it is appropriate to note here that countries differ considerably in the relationships that are possible between governmental and voluntary organizations. In English-speaking countries, for example, the aim has generally been to attain some sort of partnership whereby the completely independent voluntary organizations might receive government encouragement and, maybe, financial support to do work which, for one reason or another, the government agency cannot undertake itself. The voluntary organizations also, on their part, are in a position to make suggestions and to contribute to the government agencies' work.

It is a characteristic pattern of organization in some countries for the voluntary agencies to be composed of more or less the same people as the governmental agencies, and to pursue much the same policy under freer auspices. In other countries, the voluntary agencies, so-called, are entirely dependent upon or controlled by the government; whereas in yet other countries the voluntary bodies may be totally separate from and perhaps rather critical of the government.

In the early days of the United Nations specialized agencies there was a great deal of interchange between governmental and voluntary agencies, but in recent years, with the increasing professionalization of the specialized agencies' secretariats and the steady development of a considerable volume of precedent, it seems to have been a common experience to find a certain bureaucratic hardening in the UN agencies' secretariats, which is making cooperation with voluntary agencies less free and perhaps less fruitful than in earlier years.

2
Voluntary Action

The most concrete example of voluntary action in the mental health field is that of the voluntary mental health association. To state this is not to imply a non-recognition of the myriad acts of goodwill that are done daily by ordinary people for those who are mentally ill or disordered. But the voluntary mental health association is the only means by which the private individual can make an effective contribution to the mental health of the community.

As was noted in Volume II, the number of voluntary mental health associations in the world has increased rapidly since the end of World War II and at the time of the Study Group (1961) there were effective organizations in more than forty countries. However, of more immediate importance has been the proliferation of voluntary mental health bodies at provincial and state, county and city, and even local community level.

THE PHILOSOPHY OF A MENTAL HEALTH ASSOCIATION
In a working paper for the Study Group, Stevenson drew attention to an analysis of the philosophical foundation of a voluntary mental health association in the *Annals of the American Academy of Political and Social Science* (March 1953) and in *Mental Health Planning for Social Action* (384). Stevenson continued:

'In a democracy in which the citizen is the ultimate authority, the citizen bears certain rights and responsibilities. In a complex society, it is not possible for him to fulfill all his responsibilities. As a single person he also does not have the force to achieve his goals. However, as an active member of a voluntary citizen's organization he acquires the strength of all the members combined and can time his efforts to achieve maximum results.

'The citizen fulfills his obligations by proxy in relation to human needs which he cannot attend to personally because of lack of time and capacity. He becomes a passive member, a financial contributor, or just a moral supporter of certain voluntary agencies, in so far as they are doing what he considers a good job.

'The unit of effectiveness of a voluntary agency is the citizen member. His activation is essential. He needs to serve as a committee man, an officer, a volunteer for service, a spokesman and a delegate. If a paid executive tries to do all the tasks himself, he pauperizes the members, overloads himself and limits the society's effectiveness. It is his task to mobilize the members for action, even if to do so slows the society's movement.'

THE ROLE OF THE VOLUNTARY AGENCY
IN MENTAL HEALTH WORK

It is impossible to give a concise account of the role of the voluntary agency in the field of mental health, because, as we have shown extensively in Volume I, the nature and character of voluntary agencies vary widely from country to country. Perhaps in the majority of countries the concept of the voluntary agency is hardly understood, but where such agencies do exist they can range from organizations of extreme complexity to the poorly supported work of a devoted single individual. An example of the former, or complex, type is the National Association for Mental Health in the United States. This is an entirely independent, voluntary organization of citizens concerned with mental health in the community. It is nationwide and, naturally, geared to the federal structure of the country. Its basic unit is the local chapter, belonging to a town or a rural community. The chapters are commonly associated by counties (or, in some cases, the county is the basic unit) and grouped together into state mental health associations, which are themselves federated with the National

Association. Although, historically, voluntary mental health organizations have usually originated out of the concern of a small group of individual citizens with the plight of the mentally ill or with defective children, most of them rapidly extend their sphere of interest to embrace a wide range of mental health problems, including welfare problems of the handicapped generally, and of the socially less adequate members of the community.

This type of independent citizen organization determines its own policies for itself, and when it is sufficiently strong it can aspire to enter into collaboration on more or less equal terms with the governmental agencies. It may suggest new lines of activity for government departments that will cover areas of work hitherto neglected; and, in return, may itself undertake certain courses of action by agreement with the governmental agency, which the latter may not be able to carry out at the time for financial or practical reasons. Such voluntary organizations often jealously preserve their financial independence from the government; but in recent years in some countries they have undertaken a certain amount of work by contract with the governmental agency. This type of partnership between government and citizen, on equal terms, as independent yet interdependent agents (always provided that the prevailing political sentiment admits of such partnership), is of great potential value for the community as a whole.

National mental health associations have different styles of organization. That of England and Wales is an example of a less complex type of organization as befits a smaller, more homogeneous country where there are no federated sovereign states to complicate the task of the national government. The National Association for Mental Health, London, has a more centralized structure than its counterpart in the United States. The Association links together a number of local associations, in counties and large cities, but the individual member tends to relate directly to the London office or to the Northern Regional Office in Leeds. The Mental Health Associations in Scotland and Northern Ireland respectively are quite separate from, but maintain close cooperative relations with, the Association for England and Wales. In the United Kingdom arrangements have been worked out whereby voluntary associations can receive subsidies from the government for general operating costs, and can work under contract to the government on specific projects, while retaining full independence of action and policy-making. It is obvious that the continued existence of a working partnership between voluntary agency and government demands a convergence of view, at least in relation to the field of work. The British, like the American National Association, has as a main objective the promotion of programmes of work wherever the need is perceived, and especially in relation to areas not provided for by governmental agencies.

A number of mental health associations in other countries resemble either the American or the British pattern to a greater or lesser extent, but a third type of voluntary agency, of which the Netherlands Federation for Mental Health is an instance, has more of the character of a coordinating agency or federation. It focuses the mental health interests of a large number of social agencies, and operates as a kind of coordinating committee with the main purposes of holding conferences, providing an information centre, and infiltrating the work of its federated organizations with mental health principles.

A fourth type of voluntary agency in the field of mental health is constituted by the independent professional organization, whose members are professionally engaged in mental health work but have grouped themselves together to promote the particular interest that they serve, most commonly through the means of meetings for the exchange of scientific papers, clinical discussions, and the like. Apart from such conferences, a programme of social action is not usually undertaken. This is a common pattern of voluntary mental health organization in Latin countries. A variant of it in several countries is the university or large hospital that creates a mental health body out of its own staff, for the furtherance of social aims.

There have been instances in several countries of government departments forming an association composed of their own personnel, which enables them to take desired action on less official grounds than would otherwise be possible. A somewhat similar type of mental health agency organization is found in other countries, where the voluntary association is set up by unobtrusive governmental action. Although the mental health agency may have some appearance of independence, its officers and executive may be subject to government approval, if not nomination; and the president is frequently a high government official. The agency operates as an unrecognized but nonetheless quasi-official arm of the government. We have drawn attention to the existence of this type of organization because, although the situation is usually well understood in the country itself—where, indeed, it may be the only way in which citizens can be drawn into active work in the mental health field, no other type of organization being acceptable—it is frequently misunderstood or misinterpreted by those who are used, in their own countries, to citizens' organizations that are totally independent of government authority.

One of the structural problems facing mental health organizations of all types concerns the balance between professional and lay participation, as they are sometimes termed. Of the mental health organizations in membership with WFMH, the vast majority (although this applies less to the two largest and most complex) are run almost exclusively by professional people with very little lay participation at an executive or directorial level. The dilemma here is that, although professional domination constitutes a real handicap in attaining the objective of citizen participation, on the other hand, it is often difficult to secure professional interest and participation in an organization that is designed and set up by non-professional people. The tensions that can arise in the latter type of organization may be no less crippling than the lack of lay participation in the former.

There is an interesting example at a national level of a combination of lay and professional participation in the National Board of the Canadian Mental Health Association. The Board, which represents all the provinces of Canada, is composed entirely of lay people, mainly business executives who have demonstrated a personal concern for the work. This body is backed by a Standing Advisory Professional Committee. This structure deserves study by mental health workers in other countries to see whether it might be appropriate elsewhere; it has been found, however, in many places that a professional advisory committee with no executive responsibility tends to be frustrating to its professional members rather than useful. Again, it is very difficult for a non-professional board to digest and use advice when it has no systematic basis on which to evaluate the advice that is given to it. The two dangers in this situation are, on the one hand, that the advice will be rejected without good reason and, on the other, that the board will become merely a dependent of its advisory body. There is a strong body of opinion that it is better to attempt to weld professional and lay people into a team, rather than to segregate their functions and try to maintain a balance between them.

In a working paper, Stevenson, discussing the work of the voluntary mental health agency from the standpoint of the United States model, emphasized the need for the agency to be based on a local area. He maintains that the key to the effectiveness of this kind of body is the degree of personal involvement of the individual citizen in his own home locality; that the primary duties of the central organization are to promote the formation of local associations, facilitate exchange, give financial assistance in times of local need, and so on. The various levels of organization – local, state, federal, etc. – do not represent degrees of authority, but are divisions of labour. The local unit concerns itself with local affairs: seeking the cooperation of local mental hospitals, and of health and education authorities; undertaking a programme of public education in mental health matters; training volunteer workers; and so forth. Those who show themselves to have an aptitude for representative action can serve on a state committee, which does not have a locally based programme of action, but concerns itself with the promotion of new work in other parts of the state, and with state legislation, the operation of health and welfare services, etc. From among the membership of these state committees, those with an aptitude for nationwide affairs may perform a similar function at the federal level.

One of the weaknesses of this type of organization, as Stevenson points out, is a tendency for a hierarchical type of relationship to develop between the local, state, and national levels. Thus the local association may tend to become dependent on the others for ideas or for direction as to how to do its work, and, in return, the state and federal secretariats may conceive of their job in terms of directing rather than of initiating and advancing. When this happens there is a danger that the national executive may become so preoccupied with managing what it regards as the lower echelons that it arouses their hostility, and it may also neglect its own primary task of improving the services provided at a national level and of experimenting in new directions. The organization of finance and money-raising is liable to become the chief preoccupation at the federal level, and ideas are relegated to limbo.

Stevenson also discusses some of the difficulties and stumbling blocks that this type of voluntary mental health agency may encounter, difficulties that arise out of the attitudes of the people involved in the work. He comments:

'The field of work of the [voluntary mental health] society includes needs for progress, of varying degrees of urgency or importance. These needs can be listed as the basis for program planning. Committees can be set up to identify various needs as they relate e.g. to the mentally ill, the defective, the offender, the school child, the employee, etc. These needs should also be rated as to priority. Such a survey will reveal far more than the association can plan to do at one time. It therefore selects the things of high priority on which to focus immediate attention and money. It is at this point that the special pleader, or psychopathological member may divert the program.

'A program even after the selection of high priorities still remains to be translated into a plan of effective action. It is here that problems of internal organization of the society may cause trouble. If the staff – paid or voluntary – or committees are preoccupied with the pursuit of departmental empire building, one tends to compete with the other. A balanced strategy can be achieved only when such departments as public education, research and legislation see their function as determined by a common goal, each as a division of labor working toward that goal, and each one dependent for its success upon coordinate progress of the others.'

Stevenson points out that it is almost bound to follow that people's interest in the fields of voluntary work will relate to their personal problems and needs, or to those of their family or friends. It may frequently happen that the basis of an individual's driving concern with a particular human problem is essentially pathological, although the result may be almost entirely beneficial except for the intrapersonal stress that may be engendered. In the case of most voluntary agencies dealing with more concrete aspects of human need – as, for example, spastic children – and in other instances where it is possible to separate the origin of the concern from its objective, such pathological drives need not necessarily constitute a problem. But, in the mental health field, when the source and the objective of a pathological interest are both psychological, they may become so intertwined as to be inseparable. Thus, almost all mental health associations recruit a number of members whose drives are of a pathological type, not uncommonly of a paranoid character. These members tend to have sharply focused, narrowly defined, and highly dynamic interests that will constantly interfere with the rational programming of the whole group. It is imperative that such people be recognized for what they are, so that they are not given assignments that involve public activities or responsibility for executing projects, or, above all, any representative role.

Commonly, these psychopathological attitudes are relatively banal, perhaps little more than a strongly held prejudice. For example, certain members may make use of an agency primarily to give vent to personal feelings of hostility which lead them to look on all government servants as if the latter were of a lower order of intelligence and of less good faith and integrity than the volunteer. Alternatively, the pathological attitude of these members may be of a more authoritarian character – expressed in excessive deference to professional or governmental authority; and yet another variant may be the dependent, irresponsible, one of 'Let the government do it, it's their job'.

Another common stumbling-block to the work of voluntary mental health agencies is the egoistical attitude of members, and, specifically, their failure to see that other voluntary agencies can also be genuinely concerned with the field of mental health, even if tangentially.

The narrowness of the interests of some members, to which Stevenson has made reference, may lead the agency to neglect important fields of activity, such as mental deficiency, or the advancement of positive potential rather than emphasis on illness. This kind of situation provides grounds for criticism for opponents of mental health work, and can be a source of weakness and embarrassment.

It may be added that, just as the voluntary agency may be embarrassed or weakened by individuals who offer their services to it for pathological reasons, so it may be put into a difficult position when it attracts the opposite reaction and, also for pathological reasons, people show hostility and opposition to its work. A very great danger is that the pathological hostility of an influential citizen may result in the identification of the voluntary agency, to a greater or lesser extent, with the community's bad objects or subversive elements. Thus the hostile, phobic individual who is intensely afraid of any conscious consideration of the psychological aspects of life may project his anxiety onto the group that is trying to operate in this area. As was discussed in Volume II, there have been a number of instances where mental health societies have encountered serious difficulties through having become identified, in the eyes of a pathologically motivated opposition, with the enemies of the community.

The risk of attracting the hostility and opposition of individuals in this way can become a major consideration in respect of those items of activity of voluntary organizations that have been undertaken in subject areas too difficult, or too controversial, for government agencies to handle. At a national level, the question of sectional support of or opposition to a voluntary mental health agency, or of the favourable or hostile attention of crank groups, may not be important, except when, as may happen, a political smear becomes unfortunately attached to the agency. At a more local level it is much more difficult for a voluntary agency to keep clear of sectarian or pressure group influences, with the consequent disadvantages of incurring partisan hostility.

An example can be taken from the recent history of the mental health movement in the United States, where some of the state member organizations that have been set up as part of the nationwide spread of the movement have become involved in race and colour issues. These issues are not a problem in mental health matters at the national level, and are only rarely troublesome at a state level, but they have sometimes proved capable of wrecking a local organization. When such difficulties do arise, it is advisable to apply mental health knowledge and skills to their solution, and not merely to react by automatic reference to a principle, however fundamental. In the race question, for example, the direct application of the basic principle of anti-segregation, even with the whole-hearted support of all the members, could defeat the whole object of the agency if, as a result, the hostile feelings aroused in certain people by anti-segregation measures were to attach to voluntary mental health activity.

At the international level, these questions are even more complex. If the World Federation for Mental Health is to be truly a world organization, it must be prepared to deal with pressures – cultural, ideological, and political – similar to those encountered by the United Nations agencies. If there is to be genuine universal representation in its work, the Federation must define its programmes and state its problems in ways that are both comprehensible and acceptable to all parties and divisions of mankind, otherwise there will never be full participation. It would appear that the international non-governmental agencies are at present no more able to resolve these complex problems than the United Nations agencies themselves.

The voluntary agencies have certain advantages, however. First, they are able to engage in advance planning and to suggest action, without having to consider the level of popular support for their policies in the country or countries concerned. Certainly they have to take very careful account of cultural and ideological positions, but they do not have to court votes, give primary consideration to the financial aspects, or worry about whether their action will jeopardize their own future popularity with the electorate.

A second advantage of voluntary international agencies is that the members of their governing bodies are not representative in the same sense as are the members of boards of intergovernmental agencies. Members of the boards of voluntary agencies are there, generally, because of their own personal involvement in the activity in progress, to the furtherance of which they are expected to contribute out of their own experience. They do not operate, like government delegates, upon instructions given to them in advance at their own headquarters. The boards of voluntary agencies are therefore able to maintain a flexibility in their deliberations and a free exchange that are unattainable in an intergovernmental setting.

A third potential advantage of voluntary organizations in general – with some attendant disadvantages – is that of being able to mobilize strong sentiment for human welfare. In many countries there is a strong tradition of service to the community, whether through religious or humanitarian organizations, and many people are concerned with various aspects of human welfare. Their concerns cover a wide field – the state of the world; peace and the prevention of war; the betterment of race, labour, and international relations; the welfare of children; the protection of animal life, and so on. In most countries the effective foci on which these people can concentrate are not clearly defined, so that there is an enormous unused potential for goodwill and hard work.

The United Nations Organization has provided a focus of international interest for such people, but its aim and structure have not been such that it could make practical use of individual goodwill and energy. An example of an international voluntary organization that was remarkably successful during the 1930s in attracting to its quite restricted aims a wide range of human goodwill was the New Education Fellowship. This example is particularly instructive because a major problem facing this organization some thirty years later is how to maintain the enthusiasm of its members at a time when its rather narrowly defined educational goals have been successfully approached in so many countries.

The question of harnessing the energy and enthusiasm of members is germane to mental health societies, national and international. These societies usually include in their membership a wide variety of people whose common bond is that they are dedicated to human welfare, but whose concepts of and relationships to mental health work may differ in many ways. One asset of mental health societies that has not, perhaps, been fully exploited is that they are among the relatively few social service activities that husband and wife can join together, a circumstance that has a great potential appeal to people who feel a concern for human welfare. For example, it is a common practice in United States mental health organizations for husbands and wives to be joint members of committees.

Most mental health organizations are faced with the difficulty of making a choice between broad concerns and narrowly defined goals. On the one hand, an organization that sets itself a limited number of specific objectives may achieve all of them within a comparatively few years, and the result may be that those members who were most deeply and exclusively attached to the particular objectives – and also, perhaps, among the most active of the society's membership – will tend to withdraw their support from the organization and continue to work in the limited field, persevering with their attack on yesterday's problems by yesterday's methods. Thus the less active majority, who remain in membership, could be left without visible aims. On the other hand, in a mental health association with a broad range of interests, the majority of the members, although genuinely concerned with human welfare, may constantly be in the position of feeling that they are without defined aims, goals, or programme, and the membership is liable to fragmentation at any time on policy matters or on ideological grounds.

As a postscript to this discussion, it may be added that, in a working paper, J. R. Rees remarked on the relatively little progress that has been made by mental health organizations in the way of an effective approach to the vital problem of tensions in a contracted world society. It can scarcely be doubted that degree of tension and quality of mental health are highly interdependent, and that the principles underlying the formation of good interpersonal relationships have a special validity in this connexion. Intergroup tensions remain perhaps the primary challenge to mental health thinking in the current age.

3
The Recognition of Mental Disorder

At a time when in many countries the level of sophistication and information about mental health and illness has risen so steeply, it is very desirable that the onset of mental disorder should be recognized early and reliably. In approaching the consideration of this topic, the members of the International Study Group were keenly aware that most of them had received their original training several decades ago. They felt that there was a risk that their discussion of a developing subject like that of the recognition of mental disorder might be influenced more than they realized by outmoded concepts of the nature of health and illness, and of the processes of recovery and treatment.

The whole field of health and disease has been surveyed recently by René Dubos (2) in his book *Mirage of Health*. Dubos draws attention to the periodic changes that have taken place in the patterns of certain diseases, and relates these to various major social changes. In many countries in recent years the cultural significance of disease phenomena has been increasingly discerned, in all branches of medicine, and particularly in that of psychiatry. Because behaviour constitutes a large and vital part of psychiatric symptomatology, the early recognition of illness and the establishment of sensitive psychiatric diagnostic criteria can be achieved only in relation to a well-defined social and cultural context. This point has been emphasized by Rümke (121) in his statement that in every culture it is necessary first to find out how to identify an individual as mentally diseased; only when that has been done can one seek to determine the nature and aetiology of the disorder.

Those whose experience of disease has been exclusively in the field of somatic illness may find it difficult to accept this approach unless they constantly bear in mind the fact that the number of possible variations, within the norm, of psychological behaviour patterns is very much greater than that of somatic behaviour patterns. The range of normal physiological and anatomical variations is restricted to quite minor degrees of difference in size of organ, and in speed, quantity, and coordination of reaction patterns. Bodily homeostatic mechanisms are strong, and this fact has made it possible to reduce the great majority of different patterns of bodily disease and disorder into well-recognized clinical syndromes, that vary more according to differences in the disease agents than according to differences in constitution. The symptoms, signs, and clinical course of pulmonary tuberculosis, for example, are basically the same wherever it may be found.

In the field of psychological illness and disorder, not only are psychological constitutional variations more labile than physical, but also the disease agencies and vectors, being tied to cultural phenomena, show many more possible combinations and fluctuations at different times. This is the background to the statement that in the case of mental disorders the first task is to identify the symptoms and signs as belonging to a distinctive clinical picture; the subsequent task is to demonstrate that a significant deviation is present not only from the socially acceptable conventions but also from the culturally determined behaviour patterns in the individual's environment. Further, it is necessary to ascertain that the sick individual is unable to conform, for more than short periods, to what is regarded as normal behaviour.

It is generally accepted as a truism that the major part of the total clinical and social picture of mental illness is composed, not specifically of the manifestations of the disorder, but rather of the repercussions of the patient's behaviour in the community. Thus the patient may become separated from or in irrational conflict with his own community; or he may be rejected, abandoned, or even persecuted; and in these developments his behaviour both derives from and contributes to his position. Incidentally, such community repercussions are not confined to psychological disorders, but are liable to occur in the case of any disorder to which great fear becomes attached – a classical example being leprosy.

When we come to consider the case of single and more homogeneous social and cultural settings, and even those in which the aetiological factors have been more or less constant in recent years, current medical literature is full of instances of clinical syndromes that have changed significantly, and in some cases to a marked degree, in the course of a relatively short period.

With reference to the present-day European sociocultural contexts, Ferenczi (211) has observed, not without some irony, that 'in our day it is becoming much more rare for people to produce obvious hysterias such as, only a few decades ago, were described as comparatively widespread. It seems as if, with the advance of civilization, even the neuroses have become more civilized and adult.' La Barre (502), referring to primitive sociocultural, religious manifestations in parts of the south-eastern United States has noted, similarly:

'Freud, in fact, predicted the decrease if not the disappearance of classical hysteria as time went on, owing to the spread of lay psychological insight into the shallow defence mechanism of mere denial characteristic of hysteria. Statistically, this is evidently true in the urbanized, sophisticated North. But what constantly surprises city-trained Northern psychiatrists is that the South still has such "old-fashioned" neuroses.'

Military medical records in two world wars have shown remarkable confirmatory evidence both of the influence of cultural patterns on clinical phenomena, and of a change of clinical picture in a single culture. Ahrenfeldt (131), from a study of official records, found that, in the British army, men who broke down under stress in World War II 'tended to develop straightforward anxiety states rather than hysterical conversion symptoms (as was so frequently the case in the previous war)'. He found a great deal of supportive evidence in the records of other similar changes in symptom pattern; and he added the comment that, even in identical age groups of the male population of this particular national and cultural group, within a period of a quarter of a century, the prevalent clinical picture resulting from the stress of war had undergone a striking, clearly recognizable, and definable change.

It might legitimately be asserted that the fact that the pattern of war has itself changed, as also have methods of diagnosis and treatment of medical problems, can be taken as confirmatory evidence that the clinical picture of neurotic and mental disorder tends to be modified by changing environmental factors. Nevertheless, the medical evidence from the two world wars suggests that these changing clinical pictures may relate more closely to longer-term social trends than to immediate precipitating stress, in that, even when conditions were comparable, the morbidity statistics revealed significant differences between the two samples.

Ahrenfeldt has commented further that, when comparisons are made concerning the prevalence of hysterical or anxiety states in some specified African or Asian populations, or in Indian and West African troops fighting side by side in World War II, it is by no means certain that the mental disorders involved are aetiologically identical with, or even related to, those that occur in a Western European, e.g. British, sample exposed to the same circumstances.

Earlier, Tooth (85) had written:

'It is doubtful whether the same diagnostic criteria are equally applicable to races with a cultural background as different as that of Africans from Europeans. . . . One is . . . forced to the conclusion that there are real differences in the quality of the psychotic reactions of individuals which make it impossible to fit them into the accepted nosological framework.'

It appears to have become much more generally accepted that, in different social and cultural environments, apparently similar clinical symptoms or syndromes may have different aetiological origins and, conversely, that different clinical pictures may have a common aetiology.

Inasmuch as clinical diagnoses are still based mainly, if not entirely, on symptomatology, the whole diagnostic position remains very unsatisfactory over most of the wide field of psychiatry. Symptom-based diagnoses may have some usefulness for purposes of comparison in a single cultural setting, within a limited period of time, provided that the diagnosticians are themselves in tune with each other and with contemporary concepts. But such diagnoses are very tenuous and unsafe criteria on which to base clinical and epidemiological comparisons between cultures, or for use in cross-cultural studies generally. It appeared to the Study Group that some recent suggestions that there may be psychiatric clinical manifestations or syndromes that are more or less specific to certain cultural areas may reflect some of the confusion that results from attempting to make comparisons where no common basis exists (73, 75, 85, 565, 569).

In some countries it is considered that the number of patients suffering from the more severe, chronic forms of mental illness is decreasing, and that medical advances have appreciably reduced the incidence, course, and severity of toxic, exhaustive, and infective conditions and of their psychiatric manifestations. And not only is there evidence of change in clinical phenomena; but the attitudes of ordinary people towards mental ill health are changing also, at least in those countries where preventive and therapeutic measures have made headway. Evidence of change is clearly demonstrated in a greater responsiveness to public education in mental health; greater acceptance of the mentally ill; a more constructive and informal relationship between hospital staff, patients, and public; increasing use of the psychiatric hospital as a therapeutic community, with the aim of rehabilitation and rapid reintegration of the patient into the community; admission to hospital at an earlier stage of the illness; and more effective treatment and aftercare at all stages.

DIAGNOSTIC METHODS

After a considerable review of the literature, the Study Group agreed with the view expressed by Ahrenfeldt in a working paper that there is no evidence of an appreciable improvement, during the period 1948–1961, in the accuracy and techniques of psychiatric diagnosis, or in the methods employed in the identification of significant aetiological, social, and cultural factors. Some members of the Study Group thought that, while little or no progress has been made in reducing diagnosis based on symptoms to a more precise nosology, there has been some definite advance in the capacity to make interpretations of data within a scheme of reference, paying full attention to social factors, i.e. in interpretation of aetiology. In his paper Ahrenfeldt commented:

'Confusion reigns in the field of psychiatric nomenclature. Little indeed is known of the aetiology of mental disorders. We are, therefore, thrown back on a necessity for most careful clinical observations on which to base our diagnoses.'

The need for careful discrimination in the use of current diagnostic techniques, and for caution in the interpretation of results derived from them, may be clearly illustrated by two examples: namely, electroencephalographic and psychological tests, both of which are extensively used in clinical practice.

With the development of elaborate and highly sensitive electroencephalographs, it has been hoped that this increasingly perfected technique will prove one of the most reliable and generally applicable of methods of differential diagnosis in respect of that wide range of neurological and psychiatric disorders which it is difficult, if not impossible, to identify with certainty by existing methods. Krapf (332) has observed:

'The optimistic contention that, based upon electroencephalography, it would be very simple to distinguish between epilepsy and hysteria did not persist very long; . . . mainly because the study of the EEG in the interparoxysmal state (which is naturally predominant in practice) is often quite useless for differential diagnosis. . . . Many clinicians are pessimistic about the diagnostic usefulness of the EEG. It is, indeed, very understandable that one should doubt the value of a method which shows the same anomalies not only in clinically "classical" epileptics and in patients with attacks with completely different phenomena, but even in individuals who have no fits in the usual sense of the word. Must we not conclude that the observation of dysrhythmias in patients without any spells obliges us completely to abandon the use of the EEG in the differential diagnosis of seizures?'

Many neurologists would hold that Krapf's conclusion has gone too far, and that there are a number of aberrant rhythmic patterns shown up by the EEG on which considerable diagnostic weight can be placed. Moreover, there is no other branch of medical diagnostic technique in which greater improvements are being made, and it may be confidently anticipated that the EEG ten years in the future will be a vastly more refined diagnostic instrument than it is today.

With regard to psychological tests, there has been some recent progress in the diagnosis of, and in differentiation between, disorders of organic and psychological origin in children, particularly by the use of improved and refined projective techniques for investigating the personality of young children (412).

It can hardly be doubted that in many places the uncritical use of psychological tests is frequently resulting in misdiagnosis. An example that is currently a cause of concern has been the mistaken early diagnosis of mental deficiency, which is sometimes established from intelligence tests administered to individuals living in poor social conditions. Intelligence tests measure, without a high degree of discrimination, a number of combinations of inborn and learnt environmental and social phenomena. Many people, particularly young children who are not, in fact, mentally defective, may return very low scores if the test is inappropriate for them or if the tester does not understand the full cultural significance of the test behaviour. In this connexion, Luria has made a useful contribution (275) in differentiating between 'pseudo-defectives' and true mental defectives by methods of investigation based on Vygotsky's work on learning abilities.

The Study Group re-emphasized the need for the greatest discrimination if psychological tests are introduced into a country other than that of their origin without prior revision, modification, and revalidation for use in the different culture. The literature is filled with examples of errors in the interpretation of results, and of misdiagnosis through failure to adapt existing tests or to devise new ones appropriate to a specific cultural or social environment. There is a great need for more research in this field, and (as has been stressed by various authors) for improved tests of many kinds to meet specialized local requirements (see also 88, 497, 512).

AETIOLOGY

Similarly, there have not been extensive advances in knowledge of aetiology in recent years, although valuable progress has been made in one or two limited areas: e.g. the identification of certain significant genetic and nutritional factors, and the appreciation of a number of important environmental, cultural, and social factors.

Dubos (2) deplores the monopolization of the field of medical aetiology, during the first half of this century, by morphological, analytical, and localistic points of view. He states:

'By equating disease with the effect of a precise cause – microbial invader, biochemical lesion, or mental stress – the doctrine of specific aetiology had appeared to negate the philosophical view of health as equilibrium, and to render obsolete the traditional art of medicine. Oddly enough, however, the vague and abstract concepts symbolized by the Hippocratic doctrine of harmony are now re-entering the scientific arena.'

He further points out that

'insistence on concrete facts need not deter from acknowledging that, under natural conditions, the aetiology of most diseases is multifactorial rather than specific. By using a broadened concept of aetiology, encompassing intrinsic and extrinsic determinants of disease, the scientific physician can hope to develop a therapeutic approach that will incorporate the human wisdom and empirical skill of the traditional medical art.'

In spite of continued and determined efforts, by investigators in various countries, to establish an essential genetic aetiology of the major psychoses and neuroses for which no purely 'organic' cause has so far been identified, or to prove, for example, that schizophrenia is a virus disease, it cannot be disputed that such concepts are not supported by evidence that would stand up to even the most cursory scientific examination.

DIAGNOSTIC CHAOS

The Study Group came to the conclusion that one of the least satisfactory aspects of current mental health practice is the generally unorganized or, indeed, chaotic state of diagnostic practice and psychiatric nomenclature, even within the area of single and relatively homogeneous cultures. The absence of a generally accepted system of pathology and nosological classification makes it virtually impossible to arrive at a convention about nomenclature and classification. Thus a vicious circle tends to be set up – lack of mutual understanding about terminology hampers the systematization of pathology and vice versa, and, in addition, confusion of nomenclature means that there can be no satisfactory way of comparing diagnoses cross-culturally, which adds to the general state of chaos.

A number of authors have written about the difficulties in this field. Krapf (332) has contributed significantly to the clarification of the vague conglomeration of so-called epileptoid, epileptic, hystero-epileptic, hysterical, and other similar conditions that has made attempts at differential diagnosis in this area so unsatisfactory. Mosse (276) has complained specifically of the misuse of the diagnosis of childhood schizophrenia:

'Our cases show how erroneous dogmatic thinking may lead to contradictory therapeutic procedures. Often they are dangerous for the child. At any rate, they deprive the child of constructive social and psychotherapeutic measures. In many cases anti-convulsive medication and then ECT was recommended in the same case within a period of a few weeks. Children of all ages are being subjected to lobotomies on the same basis. Childhood schizophrenia is at present in the United States a fashionable and much abused diagnosis. Careful clinical study indicates that far more often than not this diagnosis is wrong. This is not only a threat to children living in a socially difficult milieu, but also hinders the progress of psychiatry as a science.'

In his now classical work, published in 1941, Bradley (268) stated: 'Psychoses of any sort are very rare in childhood. Schizophrenia before the onset of puberty is so unusual that individual cases are still reported as clinical curiosities.' Most psychiatrists would agree with Bradley that, by the strict criteria of schizophrenia as applied to a mental disorder in adults, it is indeed a rare condition in childhood; but, as Soddy (278) contends, it is in principle unsound to extrapolate the experience gained with what may be essentially a deteriorating disorder of the mature organism in respect of a developmental disorder of the immature. It has been clinically established that disorders of relationships are by no means uncommon among young children; what is erroneous here is, in Soddy's view, the application of a concept of an illness occurring in the mature organism.

Reviewing the discussion in this field, the Study Group affirmed that inadequate diagnostic techniques, nosological confusion, ignorance of aetiology, and uncertainty of the significance of social and cultural differences, or failure to take these into account, are major causes of misdiagnosis. The consequences of misdiagnosis or of the loose application of diagnostic labels may be seriously harmful to the patient and to the community; examples are the labelling of an individual as 'hystero-epileptic', or a diagnosis of mental deficiency for retardation due to deprivation, referred to above as 'pseudo-deficiency' (Jervis, 359).

Perhaps the most widely abused diagnostic labels having serious social consequences for the individual are those of 'psychopath', 'psychopathic personality', 'psychopathic state', etc. Ahrenfeldt (132) has written:

'A survey of the medical literature on "psychopathic personality" reduces the reader to a state of cynical despair: to one author, any delinquent is *ipso facto* a psychopath; to another, any person suffering from any form of mental disorder or, indeed, it would seem any person at all except the author concerned, is a psychopath. Definitions are innumerable and contradictory, and there is clearly little hope of agreement on this matter in the near future.'

Stengel (59) has made an important contribution to the re-establishment of psychiatric taxonomy:

'Psychiatrists have for some time paid too little attention to their diagnostic concepts which often differ considerably, even among members of the staff of the same hospital or institute. If, for instance, some psychiatrists regard recovery as incompatible with the diagnosis of schizophrenia and others do not hold this view, and if they have not made it clear to each other that their diagnostic concepts differ fundamentally, how can they be expected to agree? But apart from these difficulties, which could be considerably reduced, the reliability of psychiatric diagnosis will remain limited to those categories where no objective criteria can be employed. Diagnostic judgement often still depends on clinical symptoms about whose presence and significance in an individual case opinions may differ. But these difficulties can be overstated. The adoption of operational definitions should go some way towards reduction of disagreements on diagnosis.'

It is noteworthy that, in support of Stengel's view, the WHO Study Group on Schizophrenia (354) restricted itself to a definition of the clinical picture from which this disease might be diagnosed.

NEW APPROACHES TO DIAGNOSIS AND CLASSIFICATION
There have been a number of attempts to break the current vicious circle by adopting approaches radically different from

that of the established categories of 'classical' psychiatry. Veil (371) has suggested that a more meaningful semeiology might be based on three 'operational' criteria: emergency, dangerousness, and severity. Henri Ey, in his textbook on psychiatry (54), has attempted a new type of classification based on acute and chronic syndromes.

In respect of children, the case for a reappraisal of the diagnostic approach appears to be even more urgent. Buckle and Lebovici (283) write:

'The psychiatrist alone cannot undertake the vast task of diagnosis, and a psychological diagnosis is necessary. It is to be hoped that, in the conditions in which psychological work should be done in child guidance centres, this diagnosis will permit a better knowledge not only of the subject's mental capacity and abilities, but also of his pathogenic conflicts, the phantasies which express them, and the structure of the corresponding ego. The diagnosis cannot concern the child alone, for . . . his disorders merely reflect the dialectic of the relations binding him to his family, which are themselves the product of an environment that must be considered in its social, economic and cultural aspects. This aspect of the diagnosis is the province of the social worker. Psychiatrist, psychologist and social worker may arrive at a common diagnosis as a result of the comparison and development of their respective points of view.'

Soddy (278) has put forward a method based on what he regards as the overriding characteristic of childhood in this connexion: the fact that the organism is immature and in a state of constant development. According to his view, time and the interaction of multiple contemporary developmental tendencies are the primary considerations. He advocates a flexible diagnostic system that takes into account four items: (a) temperamental type; (b) identification of noxious factors, together with the age and stage of development of the child when these factors were important; (c) identification of the child's personal reaction patterns to stress; (d) the effect of ongoing environmental influences, including the family constellation and the interpersonal relationships of the child.

In a working paper, Levy and Goldfarb described a scheme for studying in detail the family constellation and the interpersonal relationships of the child. Taking the case of psychotic children, they put the question: 'What is there in the interactional conduct of mother and child that is a source of the deviant behaviour of the child?' They reported:

'For example, in preliminary observations, one mother constantly frustrated her child by taking his compulsive questions literally when he was using them to express a widespread and disturbing anxiety. In other words, she lacked emotional understanding of a child who, on the surface, was asking repeated questions of what appeared to her as extraneous detail. Another mother used vocabulary years in advance of her child's understanding and eluded emotional interchange as well. Another mother was uninterested when her son spoke coherently but joyously rewarded his pathological expressions of grandiosity by great approval.'

These suggestive observations raise a whole series of further questions, such as: What should be regarded as appropriate behaviour in the mother of a disordered child? To what extent and in what circumstances does the mother herself contribute to the pathological state of their interpersonal relationship?

There is wide agreement with the idea expressed above that diagnosis in the fields of psychiatry and mental health is essentially a team responsibility; and nowhere is this more valuable than in the early recognition (and early treatment) of mental disorder. There was, moreover, considerable support in the Study Group for the view that, because of the inadequacy of many existing diagnostic techniques and the general poverty of reliable scientific data in this field, exact early diagnosis is not a realizable ideal at present. This state of affairs should be a stimulus for action and research into the development of further diagnostic techniques which could, like x-rays in the diagnosis of chest diseases, for example, be applied by technicians but interpreted in the main by clinicians. Psychological tests meet this criterion to a certain extent, but that field of work has a professional responsibility of its own, not only for applying, but also for devising and interpreting the tests, for which specialized expert training is required. In this respect, then, they are not strictly comparable with medical auxiliary diagnostic techniques, which are devised by doctors and interpreted only within strict and narrow limits by technicians.

It is insisted that the personnel operating these diagnostic tests should not be asked or expected to perform the role of the psychiatrist. Their training should not be directed towards a partial knowledge of psychiatry but towards the recognition of phenomena that are of psychological, clinical, and diagnostic significance on the basis of the technical competence of the observer as the result of the application of his technique.

Discussing specifically the role of the psychologist and the legitimate use of tests, Buckle and Lebovici (283) have well stated:

'. . . at the stage of diagnosis, an important task of the psychologist is to assess the abilities of the child and those behaviour disturbances which may be measured by quantitative tests. The choice of the tests necessitates, in fact, a certain initial diagnosis. In any event, the interpretation of the tests should always be carefully studied; assessment should take into account the situation in which the child finds himself during the examination and his results. It is frequently impossible to interpret the results of the tests without knowledge of the patient's complete history, and without having discussed the case with the other members of the team. . . . The psychologist must verify his hypotheses as to the child's psychology as they emerge during the examination. Here, projective tests come into their own.'

One common criticism that is made of the effectiveness of diagnostic method can be applied with particular force to the field of mental health: there is a general lack of consonance between the information obtained by diagnostic methods and the quality of function and efficiency of the individual under observation. A psychiatrist quoted the example of an experienced airline pilot who was grounded, after many years of trouble-free flying, as a result of an unfavourable report at the latest of his two-yearly flying tests. The review of his case required that he be under observation for a period of six weeks, at the end of which time it was reported that he was fit for duty; he returned to flying for a further period of two years, with no untoward effects.

This illustration could be paralleled many times in various aspects of mental health diagnostic work. Clearly, there is a great need for the development of more reliable diagnostic and prognostic methods, not only in the mental health field, but in the whole of medical science. The problems encountered in this area are often poignant: for example, a young couple wishing to marry may seek advice if one of them has, at an earlier time, suffered some kind of mental illness or disorder, or if they fear a 'bad' (family) heredity, or are anxious about cases of mental deficiency or psychosis in close relations; or a couple may seek advice about having further children after the birth of a defective baby.

POTENTIAL DISADVANTAGES OF EARLY DIAGNOSIS
The Study Group discussed the possibility that there may be harmful consequences for the individual in the earlier recognition of those diseases to which a stigma is attached in the public mind. The diagnostician's ideal is to improve methods of recognizing a disease so that treatment can be instituted earlier and earlier in the history of the illness, in the hope of achieving a complete cure without residual disability. This ideal has been approached with conspicuous success, for example, in the case of pulmonary tuberculosis, which formerly attracted a very unfortunate stigma. However, unless the public image of the disease changes to keep pace with the improved diagnostic and therapeutic methods, the result of very early case detection may not

be an unmixed blessing to the patient. If the person whose tuberculosis is spotted at a very early stage had to go through life with the same kind of stigma that used to attach to the illness when it was detected at a late stage and almost invariably left a residual disability even if the disease were arrested, he would be paying a very heavy and undeserved penalty for medical efficiency. Ironically, he would be far worse off than scores of his fellows – perhaps the great majority, if x-ray evidence is to be believed – who suffered from a mild, undetected, and spontaneously remitting form of the disease in early childhood.

An example of harmful consequences following, paradoxically, improved diagnostic methods has been provided, until recently, in respect of the detection of minor cardiac lesions during early childhood, when public and, in this case, medical attitudes did not keep pace. This problem is now, happily, largely remedied but, up to the recent past, diagnostic evidence was accepted without due regard to functional efficiency, and public opinion continued to expect complete rest and protection for 'weak hearts', with the result that many children were treated as cardiac invalids without sufficient reason and with disastrous consequences for their psychological development.

In the field of mental illness, great advances in diagnostic methods fifty years ago led to the labelling of a large number of patients with the diagnosis of schizophrenia. At that time, the natural history of this disease was less well understood and the diagnosis of schizophrenia carried with it a more or less hopeless prognosis. Patients labelled vaguely and unspecifically as 'schizophrenics' have borne the stigma of this 'hopeless' disease for years, and although they may have fully recovered from what may have been a transient schizophrenic episode, and be emotionally, intellectually, and socially well adjusted, yet they may have been precluded from certain types of more skilled employment, or from settling and working in some other country, or, by social pressure, from marrying and establishing a family. The stigma is far worse when, as has happened very often in the past and, to a lesser extent, is still happening today, the diagnosis of schizophrenia is accompanied by some form of legal certification of insanity. Whatever may be the law about the cancellation of a certificate of insanity, the unfortunate patient will have the greatest difficulty in escaping from the slur of certification for the rest of his life, and for as long as he remains in contact with people who knew him at that time.

It appears, today, that a similar stigma is attaching to the term 'deterioration', because it is frequently being loosely applied to elderly individuals. While everyone over, say, the age of sixty must accept that he has undergone some degree of deterioration, as shown by certain anatomical and physiological signs of degenerative changes, this is a very complex field of phenomena. For the most part, people in this age group are not deteriorating to any appreciable extent in their essential functions. Indeed, the contrary may often be true because, as a result of their learning and experience, they may function not only at an unimpaired, but even at an increased level of efficiency, though they may appear to be slower and more deliberate in their reactions than younger and less experienced individuals. The Study Group concluded that great harm can be done to middle-aged people by the thoughtless attachment to them of the label of deterioration.

THE CHANGING PUBLIC IMAGE OF DISEASE

The improvement of diagnostic methods, therefore, calls for commensurate modification in the public image of disease. As we have seen, where the public image remains as it was at a time when the probable effects of the disease were much more serious, not only may earlier detection create enormous difficulties for the individual patient, but medical efforts towards still earlier recognition may be hampered if not defeated by public resistance to prophylactic measures.

In a working paper, Stoller wrote of the complexity and difficulty of eliciting the mental health problems of a population. He pointed out that rapid social change, especially with urban-rural migration, is accompanied by a considerable increase in the incidence of neurosis, delinquency, crime, alcoholism, and social distress arising out of old age and mental illness. None of these difficulties may be recognized by the general population as being within the field of mental illness and disorder, and community efforts towards their study and eradication may therefore be diffuse and imprecise. Stoller noted, further, that many problems of mental illness and disorder may be submerged, and come to light only as a result of social pressure or change – as in Thailand, for example, where mental deficiency was not recognized as a problem until recently, when compulsory education was introduced; and where opium addiction was not considered a serious matter until social action compelled addicts to register and brought to light an estimated minimum number of 100,000 addicts.

Several members of the Study Group drew attention to the likelihood that impressions of the incidence of mental disorder are often deceptive, owing to variations in case-finding opportunities. If neurosis is not recognized in the community as a medical concern, there will be few opportunities for its detection. Similarly, the identification of mental illness within the community is influenced by the way people are valued and treated as individuals, and by the degree to which social eccentricity is tolerated in the community or individuals are permitted to live without contributing to their own maintenance.

There is another and more general factor that influences case-finding opportunities, not only in the field of mental illness and disorder, but also in general medical fields and in many areas of educational and social action. It commonly happens, if it is not a general rule, that although people may be conscious of the existence of a problem that needs solving they do not bring the matter to the attention of an agency unless they have some belief in the agency's capacity to contribute to a solution. On the other hand, if the work of an agency is successful, it will lead to greater realization in the community of the realities of the problems involved, so that ordinary people are in a better position to take appropriate action when they recognize a particular difficulty.

On the whole, it may be said that the full extent of a problem is not recognized in society until the measures developed to deal with it are approaching adequacy. Thus it is often claimed that an increase in the prevalence of neuroses follows the establishment of clinical facilities for the treatment of these conditions; and it is sometimes suggested that, if left untreated, a problem would have resolved spontaneously (or, according to another view, continued to exist unrecognized in the community). It appears logical to conclude that complete recognition of psychiatric disorders in the community can be envisaged only when the public image of psychiatric disease corresponds more or less closely with the professional one.

News of a recent attempt to bring these two images closer together comes from Montreal, where a clinic has been established to which people can go for a mental health check-up. It offers facilities, in a different field, not unlike those of the well-baby clinic, to which healthy children are taken. The Montreal clinic is based on the skills of social workers, and its main purpose is to enable the client to check his own state of health. More and more, and in various countries, people are going to hospitals for a check-up on physical health. The success of such a venture depends foremost upon public attitude and it might be that, in some communities, the same result could be obtained in a rather less clinical setting by the employment of a community social worker who would be available to those who wished to take advantage of the service.

The suggestion of making provision for mental health check-ups is attractive at first sight, but it is unlikely to be very fruitful unless some way can be found of overcoming the difficulty encountered by even the most securely established well-baby clinics in the countries where these clinics have proved most successful: namely, that they are less effective in helping with the problems of those members of society who are most in need of help.

The Study Group concluded that the idea of a mental well-being clinic is a very promising one, provided that the counsellors accept responsibility to maintain a continuing relationship

·55·

with the community, to keep in close touch with what is happening there, and to be available over a sufficient period of time. This is hardly the type of work that can be undertaken in a career service with frequent changes of staff. It is only when a continuing relationship has been built up that it is safe to offer advice on human problems, and then only sparingly.

It would seem that community resources rarely stretch to provide a counselling service for all who may feel the need of help, so that attention should be focused on that section of the population which is at greatest risk; and in this connexion we would think particularly of the climacteric period, male and female, and of the period immediately preceding retirement.

4
The Modern Mental Hospital

TRENDS IN THE HOSPITAL TREATMENT
OF MENTAL ILLNESS
Since 1948, in many parts of the world, profound changes have
been taking place in hospital practices with regard to the treatment of cases of severe mental illness. Changes have been occurring in two main directions: in the legal procedures governing
the admission of patients to psychiatric hospitals; and in the
attitudes to and aims of treatment within the hospital.

The rigid legal control of admission to mental hospitals
characteristic of most European and American countries during
the past hundred years does not, in fact, date from earlier than
the mid-nineteenth century. Its origin coincided with the growing acceptance of responsibility by the community for the treatment of its mentally sick members. It is generally true that a
hundred years ago this aspect of community responsibility was
held to apply only to the more indigent who were unable to pay
for their own treatment, and it was mainly for these people that
the legal safeguards were enacted. Those who have been able to
pay their way have, in most countries, been able to obtain whatever treatment has been currently available for acute psychotic
episodes, without legal formality.

In retrospect, it appears probable that much of the horror that
has been felt, in most countries, at the idea of committal to a
mental hospital has derived from social attitudes to hospitals
intended for those who could not pay for themselves. In other
words, the shame of social failure has been added to that of
mental illness. The mental hospital, like the poor house or any
other community provision for paupers, has been looked upon as
a place to keep out of at all costs. This attitude has made it

necessary for the community to arm itself with legal powers to compel the admission of unwilling patients – a circumstance that brought in its train the need to invent forms of legal protection so that these powers could not be abused.

There have always been exceptions to the rule requiring a legal order to admit a patient to a public mental hospital. An example was the psychiatric 'emergency' service set up in the middle of the nineteenth century at the Hôtel-Dieu, the oldest hospital in Paris. Here, patients suffering from acute psychotic episodes could be admitted temporarily without complex legal procedures for 'internment' (6). During the first half of the twentieth century it became increasingly realized in a number of countries that the rigid legal control on mental hospital admissions was stifling mental hospital treatment. The movement for the emancipation of mental hospitals appeared simultaneously in several countries. In 1930 a highly significant step forward was taken in the United Kingdom with the passage of the Mental Treatment Act, which established a procedure for voluntary admission and discharge without legal certification. It is to be noted that it was necessary to introduce legislation because of the assumption there, as in other countries, that legal compulsion was an essential part of mental hospital treatment.

The rate of progress of the emancipation movement can be judged from a comment a little more than twenty years later (1953) by the WHO Expert Committee on the development of community health services (195) to the effect that its report

'presupposes legislation on the care of psychiatric illness which is based on modern psychiatric knowledge. Few countries, however, have such legislation. In many countries, voluntary admissions to mental hospitals are not provided for by law. Similarly, the commitment procedures whereby patients unwilling to accept treatment are sent to hospital, are archaic. There are in some countries, obstructions also to the provision of good psychiatric treatment, arising from obsolete laws which may, for instance, prevent females from nursing male patients or may prevent social contact between male and female patients.'

Acting on the Committee's recommendation, WHO subsequently carried out a survey of existing legislation (405) and the Expert Committee (406) commented further:

'It may be considered that at present, in almost all countries, very modern tendencies, whereby the mental patient is regarded as a member of the community in need of aid and treatment, co-exist with archaic cultural survivals, whereby he is regarded as a madman (an alienated person) whose state calls above all for measures of segregation and protection, with respect both to himself and to others. This co-existence in certain countries of very advanced laws and very primitive attitudes towards patients is very striking. Conversely, in other countries very effective psychiatric treatment and care have developed successfully, whereas the legislation reflects obsolete ideas. The conclusion to be drawn from this is doubtless that the ideas held by the masses as regards mental disease are still, even in the most advanced societies, at a very primitive stage and that legislation should, above all, encourage change in these ideas without antagonizing them in too peremptory a manner.

'To summarize, the problems raised by the treatment and care of mental patients are relatively simple. What is required is to give these patients facilities for treatment and the possibility of guardianship and medical supervision in accordance with their medical needs and social inadequacy. The different methods of solving these problems are extremely complex since they must vary according to the social structure of each country. No one system can be applicable to several different countries and in even one and the same country the systems advocated by some will be repudiated by others. Any system which comes into conflict with legal or cultural conceptions is inapplicable. It would seem, therefore, that preference should be given above all to establishing laws strongly integrated into cultural traditions while at the same time leaving the way open for possible changes.'

In the United Kingdom, the *Report of the Royal Commission on the Law relating to Mental Illness and Mental Deficiency, 1954–1957* (404) recommended

> 'that the law should be altered so that whenever possible suitable care may be provided for mentally disordered patients with no more restriction of liberty or legal formality than is applied to people who need care because of other types of illness, disability or social difficulty. Compulsory powers should be used in future only when they are positively necessary to override the patient's own unwillingness or the unwillingness of his relatives, for the patient's own welfare or for the protection of others.'

Thus in Britain a principle was laid down, and subsequently incorporated in legislation in the Mental Health Act, 1959, that completed the reverse of the legislative trend towards compulsion in treatment that had lasted for more than a century. It should be noted that this final reversal was achieved twenty-seven years after acceptance of the principle of voluntary admission. In fact, the way had been well prepared by the successful working of the Mental Treatment Act of 1930. In 1959, the last year of operation of this Act, the proportion of certified patients compulsorily admitted to mental hospitals in the United Kingdom was no more than 11 per cent of the total admissions (cf. 13·5 per cent in 1958; 49 per cent in 1946).

It is important to recognize the full significance of the United Kingdom Mental Health Act of 1959. This Act is a considerable advance on the principle of voluntary admission, which involved the signing of forms and a contractual agreement between the patient, or his representative, and the hospital. The contract has now been replaced by the principle of informal admission which, just as in the case of any other illness requiring hospitalization, needs no more than the mutual consent, which can be arrived at orally, of the patient or his representative, and the responsible doctor of the hospital.

In their study, Krapf and Moser (5) report that admissions to mental hospitals on a voluntary basis have reached more than 75 per cent of all admissions in Japan, Taiwan, the United Kingdom, and Serbia (Yugoslavia); and between 45 and 60 per cent in Ireland, Portugal, Sweden, and New Zealand. In Canadian short-stay hospitals, the voluntary admission rate is around 75 per cent; in Austria, Ireland, Guatemala, Sweden, and New Zealand 50 per cent of patients are admitted by administrative court order, and about 9 per cent in Egypt. Figures for the Soviet Union are not easily comparable, but in principle admission there depends on a medical decision. The returns cited in this inquiry (for 1960) for the United States showed that in ten states some 25 per cent of first admissions entered voluntarily. It must be remembered, however, as we have pointed out elsewhere, that in the United States patients in their first period of mental illness are more likely to be admitted to the psychiatric services of general hospitals than to the state mental hospitals. Almost all of this far bigger category of admissions is voluntary. Few general psychiatric services have authority to take patients on commitment. It is possible that the overall voluntary admission rate in the United States is no lower than that for the Canadian short-stay hospitals.

State-by-state variation of legislation in the United States, and province-by-province variation in Canada, have led many physicians in these countries to work for a standard or uniform commitment law for mental patients. In the United States, the National Institute of Mental Health formulated a model draft Act in 1950, republished in 1952 (now out of print), liberalizing admission procedures (396, 397), but this has not yet found a wide measure of public support and there is still great room for improvement in this matter.

Many of the other geographically larger countries with a federal structure have to contend with difficulties caused by discrepancies and inequalities in procedure from province to province. Again, some of these differences appear to result from various public attitudes to the free treatment of indigent patients rather than from the actual nature of the illness.

It appears that in no country is there adequate provision for even the most serious cases of mental illness, and the need for action is urgent. However, the changing pattern of mental hospital care seems to be a more immediate preoccupation in some countries and there is impressive evidence of change.

Two of the strong current trends in the United Kingdom are illustrated in *Figure 1*, which shows the variations in the size of the mental hospital population and in the mental hospital admission rates for the period 1951–59. It should be noted that the

Figure 1 Comparison of United Kingdom mental hospital admission rates and size of mental hospital population, 1951–59

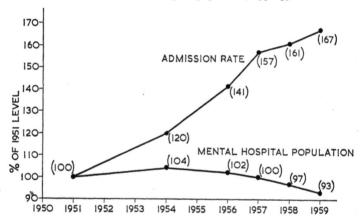

new procedure for informal admission to mental hospitals, introduced during 1959, had, by the end of that year, reduced the proportion of patients remaining in mental hospitals in England and Wales under the old compulsory form of admission to 69 per cent of the 1951 figure. It is understood, although more recent figures are not easily comparable with earlier ones owing to the radical changes in procedure, that since 1959 there has been a greater proportionate increase in informal admissions and a tendency to a far quicker turnover of patients.

In regard to turnover, the figures that are available are not very useful for purposes of comparison because of the wide variation between various hospitals, even in a single country, in treatment policies, in the stage of the illness at which patients are most commonly admitted, and in the varying longevity of sufferers from chronic forms of mental illness. Another factor complicating the statistics is that hospitals in different countries have different attitudes towards their responsibility for the rehabilitation of patients. Thus in some hospitals of the United States, for example, a patient may be carried 'on the books' of a hospital as being still under rehabilitation for as long as three years after ceasing to be an inpatient. Krapf and Moser (5) found that the average duration of stay in mental hospitals ranged in different countries from thirty to 763 days, but they noted that there has been a general tendency for the duration of stay to shorten by about one-third or more.

It would be more interesting to know the average duration of stay of patients who stay for less than, and more than, one year respectively; but these data figures are not easily obtainable. Figures relating to the United Kingdom show that nearly 90 per cent of all discharged mental hospital patients are discharged within one year. Figures for Scotland in 1958 (under now super-seded legislation) showed that the median stay of certified patients staying less than a year was about thirteen weeks, and that of voluntary patients about six weeks. For the total hospital population, the median stay of certified patients was about twenty-three weeks, and that of voluntary patients about seven weeks. Thus it would appear that comparatively few voluntary patients stay for longer than one year. It is too early yet to see the trends in the United Kingdom caused by the introduction of informal admission in 1959.

As far as the United Kingdom is concerned, the interesting fact stands out that, in the period 1951–59, although the number of occupied mental hospital beds declined by 7 per cent, the total number of admissions increased by 67 per cent. There is nothing to indicate that these striking trends will not continue; they may, perhaps, become even more marked; but there are a number of imponderables that might upset all calculations. For example, a serious trade recession or slump, or a period of economic hardship for whatever reason, might cause considerable variations in existing trends.

Between 1946 and 1956 careful estimates were made, in the United Kingdom (103) and in the United States (160, 384), of the numbers of psychiatric hospital beds and trained personnel required in proportion to population. It has been suggested that the standards used have a reasonable degree of relevance to the needs of other countries in Western Europe but, in view of the rapidly changing therapeutic conditions, this appears at least doubtful.

The WHO Expert Committee on Mental Health in 1953 (195) recommended a tentative minimum number of 'essential' psychiatric beds, 'which any country, regardless of its level of economical development, should aim to provide' for the segregation and treatment of those requiring hospitalization or 'emergency psychiatric inpatient care'. Subsequently it has become increasingly apparent that such estimates have comparatively little value, even in the countries with the most advanced and organized research and treatment facilities. Generally speaking, it is still true that the prevalence and incidence of psychiatric disorders in the community as a whole can only be guessed at. In most countries the statistics available relate only to patients who have attended hospitals or outpatient clinics; while this situation continues, the planning of hospital-bed provision must remain, to an appreciable extent, an empirical and experimental process. This is so not only in respect of the number of beds required and the use to which they will be put, but also with regard to the number and type of personnel that are most appropriate and most needed.

Thus a forecast made early in 1960 by the British minister of health that, by 1975, the number of beds in mental hospitals in Great Britain would be reduced by half has been taken with a certain amount of reserve, and the various conflicting considerations that have been aroused will be discussed more fully below. His forecast, made at the same time, that general hospitals will increasingly take over the treatment of the mentally ill, is perhaps less controversial, and there is ample evidence in the United Kingdom at least of planning along these lines.

Whatever may be the principal trends in the hospitalization of psychotic patients in the future, it is clear that in most countries the main basis for hospital treatment of mental disorder will continue for many years to come to be the separately designated psychiatric hospital. Krapf and Moser's study (5) of the number of beds in complete psychiatric hospitals per hundred thousand of the population showed, in 1959, enormous variation among the twenty-seven countries concerned:

No. of beds per 100,000 population (1959)	Country
2–49	Colombia, Guatemala, Honduras, Iran, Pakistan, Peru, Taiwan, Thailand, Yugoslavia
50–99	Brazil, Costa Rica, Japan, Portugal, USSR
100–149	—
150–199	Austria, France, Germany (Federal Republic), Israel
200–249	—
250–299	—
300–349	Australia, Canada, Finland, Switzerland, USA
350–399	UK
400–449	Sweden
over 450	Ireland, New Zealand

It seems likely that these figures reflect variations in the interpretation of what constitutes a 'complete psychiatric hospital'. Their parallel study of the increase in bed provision found that several of the countries that had fewer than a hundred beds per hundred thousand population in 1951 had increased this ratio by over 100 per cent in the next ten years; whereas most of the countries with more than three hundred beds per hundred thousand in 1951 showed less than a 20 per cent increase. The data suggest that overcrowding of beds may be a serious problem in some countries, an occupancy rate of between 110 and 129 per cent being returned by Canada, Costa Rica, Pakistan, Peru, and Thailand, and of over 130 per cent by Brazil, Colombia, and South Africa.

A pressing problem in many countries is what to do with their old-style hospitals, built to last for hundreds of years, when the costs of replacing them under new building programmes are prohibitive. There is a growing volume of experience on how to make the best use of inconvenient premises by imaginative adaptations and reconstructions and by staffing policies (64, 156, 180, 181). Nevertheless, many countries still have to contend with antiquated, gloomy, dilapidated, and grossly overcrowded buildings. These buildings might be regarded as visible symbols of the rejection of their inmates by the community. It appears to be a general rule that the more inadequate the scale of accommo- dation for mental hospital cases in a country, the more neglected and decayed the buildings and the less the readiness to improve matters. In some countries, indeed, mental patients are still in- carcerated in sections of local prisons, or in primitive and ancient fortresses, or other buildings that happen to be there and are no longer wanted for other purposes. A report to the government of one Central American country, as recently as 1957, described the mental hospital as 'dilapidated, rotted, and rat-infested', and some of the wards as 'massive fire traps' with two or more patients in some of the beds, and others 'sleeping on the bare wooden floors between or under the beds'. Conditions in many mental hospitals in Asia and Africa are not much better than this, and recent reports in India and Nigeria have drawn attention to the lack of progress in twenty years despite the fact that the in- adequacy of the conditions has long been recognized.

Therapeutic programmes as well as buildings are being criti- cized. The United States Joint Commission on Mental Illness and Health (389) reported:

'One of the most revealing findings of our mental health study is that comparatively few of 277 state hospitals – probably no more than 20 per cent – have participated in innovations designed to make them therapeutic, as contrasted to custodial, institutions. Our information leads us to believe that more than half of the patients in most state hospitals receive no active treatment of any kind designed to improve their mental condition. This is the core problem and unfinished business of mental health. Eight of every ten mental hospital patients are in state institutions. These hospitals carry a daily load of more than 540,000 patients, and look after nearly a million in a year's time.'

It is virtually certain that studies of equal candour in the United Kingdom and Europe generally would reveal a state of therapeutic inertia hardly less shocking.

In a valuable study, Greenblatt *et al.* (167) have drawn attention to the current trend of replacing old-fashioned, isolated mental hospitals by smaller specialized units, usually of about three hundred beds. Mental hospitals of larger than a thousand beds are now thought to be undesirable. Basic recommendations for the construction of small, autonomous units and also for the conversion of old buildings were made in a report to the World Health Organization (157). The Joint Commission on Mental Illness and Health (389) has recommended a policy of establishing intensive psychiatric treatment centres:

'Smaller state hospitals, of 1,000 beds or less and suitably located for regional service, should be converted as rapidly as possible into intensive treatment centres for patients with major mental illness in the acute stages or with a good prospect for improvement or recovery if the illness is more prolonged. All new state hospital construction should be devoted to these smaller intensive treatment centres.'

The Commission has also put forward a principle for the care of chronic mental patients:

'No further state hospitals should be built, and not one

67

patient should be added to any existing mental hospital already housing 1,000 or more patients. It is recommended that all existing state hospitals of more than 1,000 beds be gradually and progressively converted into centers for the long-term, combined care of persons with chronic diseases, including mental illness. This conversion should be completed in the next ten years. Special techniques are available for the care of the chronically ill and these techniques of socialization, re-learning, group living, and gradual rehabilitation or social improvement should be expanded and extended to more people, including the aged who are sick and in need of care, through conversion of state mental hospitals into combined chronic disease centres.'

SOME CURRENT PLANNING
OF PSYCHIATRIC TREATMENT

The Joint Commission on Mental Illness and Health (389) has further advocated that large general hospitals with good physical plant should be converted into rehabilitation centres for all types of chronic patient, as soon as small dispersed psychiatric units are added to them.

There is a tendency to use mental hospitals more flexibly. A good example, taken from many possible, is that of the Massachusetts Mental Health Center. This combines a teaching unit of Harvard University and a mental disease research centre of the Commonwealth of Massachusetts. There are 210 patient places: ten are for small children and are situated in a research building; the remaining two hundred are divided into four units of fifty beds each, with independent medical, nursing, and supporting personnel. Any type of adolescent or adult mental patient may be received in any unit, and can be cared for on a full-time, day, night, or part-time programme, according to need. The patient retains the same professional personnel to look after him throughout his stay in hospital, and in the aftercare programme.

Though a report of the WHO Expert Committee (390) in 1957 and a related article by Tooth in 1958 (182) both described the 'good' psychiatric hospital, they recommended, in addition, the establishment of small inpatient psychiatric units within general hospitals. They considered that the relatively small size of such inpatient units facilitates the practice of resocialization procedures, and enhances the possibilities of liaisons with other medical and social community services.

We have referred above to some impressive evidence of change in mental hospital statistics. In a working paper, Buckle (656) has examined the fact that the length of stay of patients in mental hospitals in the United Kingdom is shortening. He regards this trend as being due to a combination of factors: the lessening severity of the cases, earlier treatment of better selected and better screened patients, better treatment, and a tendency to discharge patients more readily; in his view it is not, at any rate substantially, due to better aftercare services. Buckle finds that his opinion is widely shared by psychiatrists in the United Kingdom, and it is also supported by the fact that hospital personnel staff are not markedly increasing in number. It is the rapidly rising readmission rate (174, 347, 351) that is considered by some to be alarmingly high and suggestive of a certain ruthlessness in promoting discharge. But an alternative opinion is often expressed: that it is better in the long run for the patient to be repeatedly readmitted to hospital and have more frequent periods of open social life than to remain for a long time in a hospital environment which has ceased to have therapeutic significance for him. Buckle points out that the current changes in policies of admission and discharge in the United Kingdom have taken place in an era of relatively high employment, when provisions for the employment of the partially disabled are protected.

Brown (347) has commented pertinently:

'While the length of stay in hospital can be studied in its own right, most find it of interest as a simple and reliable criterion of outcome. This view has considerable justification since discharge is undoubtedly highly related to clinical improvement in schizophrenic patients. However, it is probably only the minority of patients who leave completely symptom-free and many will be re-admitted. With the decreasing use of certification these trends are likely to become, if anything, more marked . . . It is now possible that re-admissions have disproportionally increased due to the discharge of more patients with a poor prognosis.

'While the possession of definite schizophrenic symptoms can co-exist with satisfactory social achievements, such as remaining in employment or a tolerable role of social dependence, former patients can be a considerable burden to their families and acquaintances. At times the suffering they cause is severe, an experience frequently undergone with little support from social agencies. Studies give no cause for pessimism about the social adjustment which discharged patients can achieve; but to-day there seems less justification for using discharge as a criterion of successful outcome without study of its wider implications. . . . Discharge is a social process in which the patient's clinical condition is only one, even if the most important, factor.'

The changes in mental hospital figures in the United Kingdom were the subject of a further statement by the British minister of health (631) in 1961. He, as noted above, had forecast in 1960 that in fifteen years' time the number of hospital beds required in England and Wales for the treatment of psychiatric patients might well be reduced by half; and that the remaining cases ought, for the most part, to be treated in wards or wings of general hospitals. The view was subsequently incorporated in a ten-year hospital plan for England and Wales (186, 188), but was criticized in many professional quarters (149, 174, 309). Hargreaves et al. (309) remarked that it had been assumed in the report that within the next thirteen years it would be possible to close 45 per cent of the existing psychiatric beds – an assumption based on a paper by Tooth and Brooke (183) – but there had been several further studies (134, 158, 170, 171) which cast grave doubts on its validity. In their opinion, another doubtful assumption was that the number of geriatric beds in the country was adequate at present. They pointed out that if either of these assumptions proved wrong, a really chaotic situation might arise. Barr *et al.* (158) reached the following conclusion:

'It is possible then to argue that two of the main factors contributing to shorter hospital stay (i.e. the use of tranquillisers, and a possible increase in the amount of accommodation) may be only transitory in their effect, and this together with the knowledge that the resident mental hospital population, although declining, has still far to go, should act as safeguards against incautious optimism. There is also the point . . . that the proportion of patients now becoming chronic shows little reduction. On the other hand even a slow trend, if it persists, will go a long way, and if new hospitals have to be built they must presumably be built with the intention in mind that they will last some fifty years. Whether or not on general grounds it seems that limits lie immediately ahead and that the gradual shortening of hospital stay will soon come to an end, it seems imperative to continue to study the current critical trends very closely.'

Another striking modern trend, which was not specifically taken into account in the British ministry of health forecast, is the very considerable rise in admission rates to psychiatric hospitals in England and Wales. In the twenty-five years from 1929 to 1954 the admission rate increased three and a half times and, as *Figure 1* shows, by another 14 per cent in the subsequent five years. T. P. Rees (147) has observed:

'Fortunately the numbers remaining in our mental hospitals have not shown a comparable increase, but as most of our mental hospitals are grossly overcrowded, it is difficult to state with certainty whether this is due to lack of beds or to improved methods of treatment.'

A factor that has helped to keep down the numbers of patients in mental hospitals is the decrease in the numbers of long-stay patients, as reported both in the United States and in the United Kingdom. This decrease was ascribed by Brill and Patton (214) to the introduction in hospital practice, after 1954, of psycho-tropic drugs. In a written communication Stevenson has re-marked that in an effort to increase the number of discharges some hospitals have tended to lower their criteria of successful therapy; thus the increased discharge rate of hospitals may look like therapeutic success. He observes, however, that this practice may not be wholly a disadvantage, because it may save patients from suffering the antitherapeutic effects of a poor hospital. Norton (174) has expressed the view that the present trend

'will involve a continually larger admission rate, a more rapid turnover of cases, and the development of psychiatric care for a wide variety of conditions which at present are received in our hospitals but accorded relatively little attention. Society has many unmet needs in this area, and the mental hospitals have a responsibility here. At the present time the New York statistics and the New York experience indicate that the unmet needs may outrun the prospects of new available mental hos-pital space, failing some revolutionary therapeutic advances.'

On the assessment of what may be the future need for psychiatric beds, he notes: 'It would seem that a very conservative attitude is justified. So far, we have not heard of a single instance where psychiatric beds were no longer able to be utilized.'

The Study Group concluded that the figures presented above showing trend in bed occupancy, admission rates, and length of stay, although impressive, cannot be used at present with con-fidence in planning for the future, because they have appeared so suddenly and so relatively recently that what may happen in the immediate future is hardly predictable. On the other hand, it cannot be doubted that the number of occupied beds in the United Kingdom, for example, is steadily going down and, since probably not more than half of the psychiatric hospitals in the country are fully involved in modern therapeutic techniques, it may legitimately be inferred that, as every hospital becomes fully up to date, and allowing for new discoveries yet to be made that will lead to still greater efficiency in treatment, the decline in the rate of bed occupancy may well accelerate.

An interesting finding in the Krapf and Moser study (5) is that of the relatively low cost of maintaining patients in psychiatric hospitals as compared with general hospitals. Of eighteen countries reporting, the costs for psychiatric patients were roughly one-quarter of those for general hospital patients in eleven countries, roughly one-half in seven countries, and roughly three-quarters in one country. However, these figures need correcting in view of the relatively greater number of chronic patients in psychiatric hospitals, which means that costly diagnostic procedures are required less frequently. United Kingdom figures show that, although mental disorder takes between 40 and 50 per cent of all hospital bed accommodation, it accounts for only 3 per cent of hospital admissions. Again, it would appear desirable to carry out some studies of hospital costs corrected by number of admissions and length of stay. Of particular interest would be further studies of the relative costs of feeding patients, along the lines of those already undertaken in some countries.

THE PSYCHIATRIC HOSPITAL AS A SMALL SOCIETY

The concept of the mental hospital as a therapeutic community, or, in other words, the idea that the social environment provided by the hospital can itself be used to great advantage for therapeutic purposes, has been increasingly accepted since the original work of Main and his colleagues (131, 192, 206) with British military patients during World War II, and its subsequent application and development in England and elsewhere (140, 163, 184, 190, 191, 194). T. P. Rees (147) has reminded us that:

'The role of the patient as an active member of the hospital team, promoting his own recovery through his contribution to the work of the hospital as a whole, brings us to the concept of the mental hospital as a therapeutic community, as an instrument of treatment in its own right. We, as doctors, are apt to flatter ourselves by attaching undue importance to specific methods of medical treatment. . . In spite of the great advances in scientific methods of treatment in recent years, perhaps the most important change from the patients' point of view has been the return to moral treatment. This is particularly true of the long-term patient in the mental hospital.'

In this connexion, the WHO Expert Committee on Mental Health (195) stated:

'The most important single factor in the efficacy of the treatment given in a mental hospital appears to the Committee to be an intangible element which can only be described as its atmosphere; and in attempting to describe some of the influences which go to the creation of this atmosphere, it must be said at the outset that the more the psychiatric hospital imitates the general hospital, as it at present exists, the less successful it will be in creating the atmosphere it needs. Too many psychiatric hospitals give the impression of being an uneasy compromise between a general hospital and a prison. Whereas, in fact, the role they have to play is different from either; it is that of a therapeutic community. As in the community at large, one of the most characteristic aspects of the psychiatric hospital is the types of relationship between people that are to be found within it. The nature of the relationships between the medical director and his staff will be reflected in the relationship between the psychiatric staff and the nurses, and finally in the relationship not only between the nurses and the patients, but between the patients themselves.'

Bierer (133) has commented that 'there is a tremendous source of therapeutic potential in the patient himself', which can be consistently and scientifically mobilized; 'by making him a fully fledged partner in his treatment, and also in the treatment of his fellow sufferers', the whole therapeutic approach to the psychiatric inpatient can be revolutionized.

In a report to the Department of Mental Health of Massachusetts (1960) on psychiatric practice in Europe it was suggested that the most significant difference between mental hospitals in the United States and in Europe generally was the greater respect for the individual shown in the latter. The writer remarked: 'It might have been expected that in the USA where individual freedom is a revered condition, this attitude would have been reflected in mental hospital care.' A similar attitude can be seen in a report on European mental health services to the Veterans' Administration (64):

'Most laudable is the concept of the maintenance of the human dignity of the individual. We believe that this . . . is a factor of great importance in the successful programmes we observed and in the maintenance of an open hospital. The consideration for the dignity of the patient, the attitude of treating the mentally ill as "just another sick person", has contributed to an effective, therapeutic doctor-patient relationship in which the patient looks to the doctor for his treatment on the same basis that he would in a general hospital and, apparently, follows the instructions as he would in that situation. This also contributes to good mental health in the community.'

The value of considering the psychiatric hospital as a social institution, and of understanding the interpersonal relationships within it, has been emphasized by Stanton and Schwartz (193). This study of 'institutional participation in psychiatric illness and treatment' draws attention to the influence on therapy of interpersonal tensions within the hospital. The authors show that in such a society collective disturbances in the ward may be related to tensions among the staff. They also show how readily tensions can mount within a system of 'blocked mobility', wherein promotion across the boundaries between the various groups – patient, orderly, nurse, ancillary staff, lay administrator, and doctor – is virtually impossible. Thus it is now being realized that the influences other than pharmacotherapy or psychotherapy that are bearing on the patients' recovery or relapse are very important indeed, and that much more attention must be turned to the 'other twenty-three hours' when the patient is not seeing his doctor.

More recently, as part of the increasing interest in this aspect of psychiatric inpatient treatment, a social anthropologist, Caudill (189), in the United States, has shown how role, status, and group-influence among patients in a small psychiatric hospital affect the course of an illness. He shows that the ability of a person to fill a relatively passive patient-role and to do well in hospital does not necessarily indicate that he would do well outside. Staff need to be aware of their relationships with each other and to examine their motivation towards the patients. Caudill concludes that, for a truly therapeutic community to emerge, drastic changes in structure are needed, and much retraining of staff. He suggests that one way out of the present tight vertical structure of hospital roles – which is, indeed, being increasingly advocated and practised in various countries – would be to encourage 'lateral echeloning', for example by permitting doctors and other staff members to undertake extramural activities, and patients to go out to work.

In countries where there are active developments in mental health work, there is increasing recognition of the value of psychiatric (interdisciplinary) teamwork for therapeutic success (167, 243, 390). The advantages and possible limitations of such teamwork, with special reference to child guidance work in different cultural situations, have been discussed by Buckle and Lebovici (283). Referring to the development of the therapeutic milieu of the psychiatric hospital, Buckle (656) makes the point that, with increased awareness of the need to modify the human relationships of the patient and, consequently, with the application of better techniques of relationship on the part of the hospital staff, relationships between the patients themselves have been brought more to the foreground. The deliberate structuring of social groups within hospitals is now a common practice, and many forms of occupational and recreational therapy are seen as essentially milieu therapies. In many hospitals, patients have been brought to an increased understanding of their own disorders through discussion groups – ranging from ward discussions led by nurses to professionally conducted therapeutic groups – which focus on their feelings and attitudes within the hospital society itself. In some hospitals, patients are, in fact, managing their own wards. The application of these techniques has done much to reduce the tendency to chronicity in long-stay patients.

The present policy of active resocialization has both preventive and therapeutic aspects. Modern techniques of introducing patients to the psychiatric services include the aim of preventing desocialization. Techniques to avert institutionalization, or 'institutional neurosis', have been described, for example, by Barton (328), who advocates an ascending 'social' scale, from patients working in groups to patients working part-time, and then full-time, with remuneration, outside the hospital, and attending social clubs, living in hostels, and so on. The hospital staff are taught how to correct the various factors that contribute to institutional neurosis, and *all* their actions with patients are directed towards an increase of contact with the outside world, reduction of hospital-enforced idleness, an absence of dictatorial authority, and an optimistic plan for discharge (cf. 352).

Alterations to the material environment in the hospital, and the fusion of occupational therapy and rehabilitation procedures, are aimed directly at returning the patient to an open community. In the past, occupational therapy given with 'diversional' aims, to supply the advantages of a hobby, frequently did not prove of therapeutic value. However, certain forms of occupational therapy based on active work patterns have now evolved, which have a stronger individual psychotherapeutic element.

The employment of chronic psychotic and mentally defective patients of even quite low grade in process work, on contract and for remuneration, is becoming useful in its extension as a method of active therapy. It is of particular value as a staged and individualized process of retraining and resocialization, having significant connexions with special workshops outside the hospital, and maintaining relationships with medical rehabilitation and retraining centres in the community. The use of tasks realistically related to future employment possibilities draws attention to the need for facilities for part-time work outside the hospital for in-patients, and for patients in aftercare hospitals and night hospitals, and also to the need for sheltered workshops adequately protected by legislative provision.

A further aspect of the resocialization trend is the development of social activities within the hospital, and their extension to social clubs, set up in the community, for patients and ex-patients (133).

THE OPEN-DOOR PRINCIPLE

One of the most significant advances in the treatment of patients in psychiatric hospitals has been the introduction and spread of the 'open-door' principle. This has both arisen out of and contributed to the development of the concept of the hospital as a therapeutic community. Medical historians have established that the open door is no new theory but has been introduced and lost sight of again at various times and in various places. Its recent reintroduction appears to have sprung from a pioneer move in Melrose, Scotland, where an entire hospital became unlocked. The principle has spread so widely throughout the United Kingdom that it is now accepted there as standard practice. Though it is not possible to state exactly what proportion of wards are entirely open in United Kingdom hospitals, it is probably an accurate summing-up of the position to say that the whole hospital is, in principle, unlocked, but that there are certain wards, not more than one-fifth of the total, which from time to time, as circumstances demand, may be locked for shorter or longer periods. It is to be noted that the successful operation of an open-door ward depends on the quality and availability of staff, and it is the staffing factor, more than any other single factor, that is limiting the universal application of this principle in the countries in which it has been adopted. Krapf and Moser (5) observe that wherever the open-door system has been introduced it has subsequently spread very rapidly, and only in strictly localized instances is there evidence of a return to locked doors. There have been encouraging reports of hospitals, in Ruanda Urundi and in Taiwan, for example, being newly constructed and run from the outset on an open-door basis.

On the other hand, in a number of countries, for example, Germany, little or no use of the open-door system is reported. And in the Soviet Union the principle is understood to mean a régime in which the patients are free to move inside an enclosed establishment, or what might be described as a hospital compound, with no closed-door isolation blocks.

It is within the hospital experience of most psychiatrists that certain patients ask to be prevented from committing destructive acts that they sense or fear they may be going to do. The Study Group noted that there has been no little confusion of thought on the question of various forms of restraint and the open-door principle. It is legitimate to regard tranquillizers, when effective, as a very potent form of chemical restraint, and leucotomy (lobotomy) as surgical restraint. It follows from this view that when a patient is violent and destructive it is a pragmatic rather than a moral question whether he is given a tranquillizer, surgery, or a form of physical restraint – a locked door, a padded room, or something more subtle, such as a continuous bath. Current literature reports that some patients fear the open-door system, and feel much more secure when there is a lock between them and the outside world. This therapeutic aspect must be taken into consideration before it is insisted that, for the sake of a principle that works well in the majority of cases, no patient shall be given the security of a locked door.

It was awareness of this aspect that led Repond, at the Maison de Santé de Malévoz, when converting an old hospital building into a modern therapeutic community, to redesign one wing to provide an internal courtyard or patio laid out as an attractive garden, where patients could be out of doors in the summer if they wished, but with a sense of complete security. And the need for security is illustrated in the remark of a patient, who had been treated for a year at one of the foremost therapeutic communities in the United Kingdom, conducted on psychodynamic lines, about 'that dreadful permissiveness'. It is evident that the

79

so-called liberal tendencies in modern mental hospital therapy, no less than all other tendencies in treatment, must be considered in relation to the needs of the individual patient.

It has even been said of some mental hospitals in Europe that they are so anxious to build up a reputation for freedom and permissiveness that they refuse to take the more difficult patients. If this statement is true, and it is hardly susceptible to proof, there would, in fact, be something to be said for the policy from the hospital's point of view. With the lessening of means of mechanical restraint in a hospital, including locked doors and a rigidly enforced code of patient behaviour, the hospital's capacity to promote a permissive atmosphere depends on the suitability of buildings and on an adequate supply of staff members who are competent to be responsible for patients' safety under the conditions of freedom that are introduced. The therapeutic community is bound, in self-protection, to be discriminating about admissions, because the presence of three or four very difficult patients in one small therapeutic group makes the task of the whole impossible. The conclusion may be drawn that the success of liberalizing tendencies in mental hospitals depends primarily on the careful selection of patients and their allocation into appropriate units.

In the course of his exploration of the potentialities of the psychiatric hospital as a therapeutic community, Main (173) undertook the imaginative and successful experiment, at Cassel Hospital, England, of admitting young children with their mothers, when the latter were in need of psychiatric inpatient treatment. Main writes:

'Now that most paediatric hospitals and wards encourage mothers to visit their children, or even admit the mother with the child, it seems odd that so much less attention is paid to the disruption in this same mother-child relationship when it is the mother who has to go to hospital.

'In this country – though not in some others – a mother admitted to hospital is usually cut off from contact with her children, whether she wants it or not. In some hospitals it is not thought proper for children, and especially young children, to go to see their sick mothers even on visitors' day. The reasons vary. . . . Such reasons are based on the partial truth that children are a nuisance; but others are based on a different half-truth – that the children will be harmed. . . .

'No one would deny that for many situations these two arguments are valid; but when applied to *all* hospitals they recall the hostile ratiocinations common a few years ago when it began to be generally mooted that the child in hospital should have frequent visits from its mother. These, too, were always logical, but they underestimated the importance of the child's relationship with its mother to its mental and physical health. . .

'We started admitting children at a time when we were experimenting with the hospital community, to see whether it could become less of a social vacuum – more a place of treatment and less of a retreat from the stresses and strains of domestic and industrial life to which the patient must inevitably return. Just as it seemed important to keep a man patient in touch with his job and to treat him for the difficulties he might meet there, so it seemed important that a mother should be kept in touch with her job, and the children who were part of it.'

Main pointed out that this hospital did not admit chronic cases, nor those under certificate suffering from gross psychoses, and that some cases would certainly be encountered in which the child would be better separated from the mother. He added that some patients needed psychotherapy before their anxiety was sufficiently allayed to enable them to receive and care for their children. He nevertheless felt that the results of this courageous experiment justified the following conclusions:

'But what has been impressive is how much can be achieved with these women. Some of our mothers have been certified in the recent past and many had been in mental hospitals. Many had found mothering an impossible task and either they or their husbands had sought foster-parents for their infants. In

81

the hospital severely disturbed, terrified, depressed, or impulse-ridden women became able to mother their children with increasing mutual benefit, and eventually to help other mothers and children.

'I would add that psychiatry needs opportunities to study severe disturbances of the mother-child relationship. Much has been written about the psychology of women, and also of infants, but remarkably little on mothering and its disturbances; and most of what has been written is concerned with the baby's needs rather than the mother's. Perhaps this is partly because it is our usual practice to separate mother and child when there is an acute disturbance of mothering. Admitting mothers and children to psychiatric hospitals may therefore be an important development for the study of these disorders.'

5
The Hospital as a Therapeutic Agent

SOME NEW TRENDS IN INPATIENT THERAPY

Where it has been introduced, the concept of the therapeutic community is causing a radical change in the atmosphere of psychiatric hospitals. The new-found freedom from restraints and the active participation by patients in their own treatment programmes have enabled a considerable breakthrough in the application of psychotherapeutic techniques to hospital life.

Many interesting developments in psychotherapeutic techniques and their use in regard to specific problems in different countries are described in a valuable series of volumes edited by Masserman and Moreno (213) and published during the years 1956–60.

On the whole, these new techniques are largely concerned with the application of the psychodynamic approach to treatment. It is obvious that the numerical factor of the therapist-patient ratio must make direct individual psycho-analysis for mental hospital patients a practical impossibility on a large scale, and it seems that the role of psycho-analysis in this connexion is necessarily limited to research purposes and the acquisition of knowledge. However, it has become evident from the development of the hospital therapeutic community in many areas that there has been quite a widespread application of psychodynamic principles to group processes which, through its effect on the social and community life of the hospital as a whole, is proving a valuable treatment aid. More specific projects of group therapy are being undertaken in many places.

One of the most encouraging aspects of current therapeutic advance has been the integrated development of physical and pharmacological treatment with psychotherapeutic and dynamic approaches. Although mutual antagonism between the practitioners of these various methods persists in a number of places, in others an increasingly collaborative attitude is appearing. Excluding this recent integrated approach, the general position regarding therapeutic measures for psychiatric inpatients has been very adequately described by Linn (243). There have been no appreciable innovations in this field between the publication of his work (1955) and the time of writing.

PHYSICAL AND PHARMACOLOGICAL METHODS

With regard to physical and pharmacological methods of treatment, Ahrenfeldt commented in a working paper:

'It is probable that the most significant new development in psychiatric therapy in recent years has been the introduction into clinical practice of the so-called "ataractic" or "psychotropic" drugs in ever increasing numbers, and with a most confusing diversity of nomenclature, as of specific effects and side-effects.

'Linn (227) has rightly drawn attention to the importance, in evaluating the effect of these drugs, of assessing such factors as environmental, socio-economic and cultural determinants and variables, "psychological tolerance", etc.

'These drugs, frequently used in association with other forms of treatment, have been the subject of most favourable reports as to their value in securing better cooperation and accessibility on the part of many patients; facilitating and accelerating the (symptomatic) recovery of psychotic inpatients; the length of their stay in hospital, and the general discharge rate (214); and they have similarly been reported to be highly effective, in the community treatment of such patients after discharge from hospital, in reducing the frequency of their subsequent visits to outpatient clinics, and assisting them in their social readjustment (217). Administratively convenient as this may be, it is important to record that some authors, while readily conceding the auxiliary value of these remedies when properly employed, have nevertheless come to regard with concern the

84

effect of such drugs on patients in mental hospitals. Thus
Sands (178) observes that "as time moves on, we are beginning
to find that patients continue to relapse and return to hospitals
as before, or that many remain in their communities but are
unable to adapt adequately even though their more disturbing
symptoms are no longer present. The result has been to turn
loose a large number of patients who are not acceptable to
their communities, their families, the hospitals nor to themselves." '

The psychotropic drugs, and in particular lysergic acid diethyl-
amide (LSD), have been used with apparent success by Sandison
(231, 232) in modified individual and group psychotherapy. But
Sandison has also made some pertinent critical comments concerning the assessment of the value of pharmacotherapy in
psychiatric practice. He observes that most clinical trials lead to
results unduly favourable to the drugs being tested, for the following main reasons: failure to estimate accurately the spontaneous improvement rate of a similar group of patients; inadequate methods of measuring improvement, which are
susceptible to conscious or unconscious bias on the part of the
observer; and the fact that trials are influenced by the 'placebo'
response. He emphasizes the need for more research, and for
improved methods of trial and evaluation of results:

'First, the pressure from drug manufacturers on clinicians
to carry out *rapid* clinical trials should be resisted at all costs.
The patients should be on placebos for weeks or months before
the drug is introduced. Before a controlled clinical trial is
carried out, the staff should learn how to use the drug and get
some idea of what can be expected of it. The editors of medical
journals should insist that authors have used the drug for at
least a year before their paper is accepted for publication.
Secondly, the first few clinical trials at any one hospital must
be regarded with suspicion because of the placebo response.
Thirdly, group meetings must be held in wards where clinical
trials are going on, and the attitude of the staff and patients

H   85

towards the trial must be ascertained. All the uncertainties and errors in clinical trials at mental hospitals or out-patient clinics lie within the emotional lives of the staff, and the operating factors should be clearly stated. The size, training and personality of the staff must be assessed, the daily lives of the patients studied, the frequency of parole and leave, etc. compared. How these factors can be assessed is difficult to say, and whether anyone would accept the loading of the results according to the group situation in the ward is doubtful. Nevertheless, until more objective studies of the social factors surrounding a clinical trial are published alongside the clinical results, data will be lacking on the real efficiency of the drugs, and psychiatry will continue to be bewildered by an alarming confusion of new drugs.'

Indeed, as Sandison (232) rightly points out:

'The most favourable results of clinical trials are obtained in backward hospitals or in wards where little effort has been made to resocialize the patients. In some mental hospitals . . . nearly all the social benefits achieved elsewhere by ataractics have been produced by group therapy, and the advocates of the open-door system and rehabilitation claim that drugs are unnecessary.'

Certain psychotropic drugs, principally imipramine (220, 229), have been used increasingly in recent years in the treatment of depressive states. But, while these particular drugs indicate a promising line for further research and development, and have proved of significant value (often in place of ECT) in certain types of depression, they have so far unfortunately been found to be less effective in the treatment of those depressive conditions that are most frequently encountered in clinical practice.

In view of the increasingly widespread use of these pharmaco-therapeutic agents, and their current prominence in the everyday life of individuals in every part of the world, the Study Group felt that it would be valuable to give some attention to the various psychiatric, social, and cultural aspects of this situation.

The members thus considered the therapeutic limitations, as well as the advantages, of psychotropic drugs in clinical practice, their abuse in certain respects, and their possible impact on the individual and society in different cultural contexts.

It has been commented elsewhere (21) that the Study Group, while drawing attention to the potential value of these drugs in facilitating the introduction of psychiatric services in newly developing countries, also stressed that would-be users should be warned against any uncritical and dogmatic acceptance of such therapeutic methods. Some of the drugs in common use have been administered somewhat indiscriminately, overestimated as to their value, and insufficiently tested – quite apart from the fact that there has been no attempt to investigate their suitability for use in different cultural contexts. Indeed, some of the methods exported to other countries have subsequently proved to be but a temporary fashion in their country of origin, where they have sometimes been abandoned even before they have been fully introduced to the new country.

There was general agreement in the Study Group on the need to scrutinize our concepts of the nature of the processes of recovery and of therapeutic intervention. In his review of the subject of treatment over a wide medical field, Dubos (2) has referred to the succession of 'fashions', in the first half of this century, for allegedly highly specific sera, drugs, etc. He observes that, whatever the nature of the disease, the primary aim appears to have been 'to discover some magic bullet capable of reaching and destroying the responsible demon within the body of the patient'. Although there are a few diseases that can be related, in greater or lesser degree, to a specific, rather than a multi-factorial aetiology, pathology, and therapy, Dubos's statement is still valid in respect of the vast majority, viz.:

'It is the responsibility of the physician to decipher the relative importance of the various factors involved in the response of each individual patient, and to decide which aspects of the internal and external environment can be safely manipulated for the purpose of treatment.'

It is still insufficiently realized by students of medicine, nursing, or social work (or, indeed, by their teachers) that treatment is specific only in a small minority of patients. In recent years, however, scientific drug trials, by their demonstration of the placebo effect, have begun to spread a healthy scepticism about specific therapy. This 'healthy scepticism' is not new. It has been a great controlling and motivating force in the development of medical science and practice, but it has been restricted to a comparatively small number of scientists. The recent spread of scepticism is but a revival of an essential principle in medicine, which had been neglected and then forgotten. Some years ago, a most eminent Scottish physician, the late Sir Robert Hutchinson, wrote (221):

> 'I am glad to see . . . that the abuse of modern remedies (and their cost) is beginning to be recognized; but I think there should be a new petition in the litany to be read in hospital chapels or wherever doctors and nurses do, or ought to, congregate. It might be as follows: "From inability to let well alone; from too much zeal for the new and contempt for what is old; from putting knowledge before wisdom, science before art, and cleverness before common sense; from treating patients as cases, and from making the cure of the disease more grievous than the endurance of the same, Good Lord, deliver us." '

But scepticism, however healthy, is not enough by itself; and the effect on the processes of recovery of the patient's emotional relationship with his physician and his nurse has so far been the subject of little, if any, scientific study.

Several members of the Study Group strongly advocated that greater effort should be made, notwithstanding the incompleteness of current information, to evaluate particular forms of treatment, even on the basis of transient phenomena. They pointed out that new drugs can be and are being used too early and too freely, before they have been thoroughly tested and proved, and they believe that legislation may assist in setting ethical standards and stabilizing community attitudes towards these drugs. There are many difficulties and potential dangers: for example, even the exploitation of the placebo effect in clinical trials can have various undesirable consequences on social attitudes to treatment. The widespread use of bromides, barbiturates, and anti-depressive and other drugs has provided evidence of a variety of psychosocial disorders within the community which are only too readily 'exploitable' by indiscriminate and popularly accessible pharmacotherapy. Indeed, in some areas where psychiatric services are underdeveloped, the dangerous concept has emerged that drugs could be a substitute for the more specific management of individual maladjustment. Drugs are undoubtedly of value as temporary agents in assisting the readjustment of the patient and his re-establishment in his society, but, however useful their contribution, they should not be overvalued.

Many doubts have been expressed on religious and ethical, as well as psychodynamic, grounds as to the implications for the individual and society of the potential effect of psychotropic drugs on the personality. A clergyman in the Study Group remarked that these doubts are commonly expressed in the form of anxiety, felt in many circles, lest the indiscriminate use of drugs by those working in the field of mental health should lower the threshold of the patients' standards of ethical responsibility. He added that it would be helpful if religious groups could be reassured or informed on this point.

A psychiatrist observed that psychiatry should be as concerned with the effect of these drugs on what might be called the 'moral' personality of the patient as with their effect on the whole psychological personality, and especially with how they may affect the individual's ability to meet his problems. The Study Group thought that Pope Pius XII, in his address to the International Congress of Psychopharmacology in Rome in 1958 (235), was expressing views held by very many psychiatrists of different schools of thought and religious belief:

'It is the whole personality which must be treated, and it is necessary to restore the instinctual equilibrium indispensable for the normal exercise of its freedom (of decision). It would not be without danger, to conceal from the patient his personal problems by providing him with relief of a purely external kind and a superficial adjustment to social reality.'

The great majority of professional people in this field agree that drugs do not in themselves provide an answer to problems of psychiatric illness or disorder, and that such problems are dependent primarily, for their ultimate solution, on more broadly-based clinical rather than narrowly pharmacological treatment.

It may reasonably be forecast that, as drugs become pharmacologically more effective (as they certainly will), the problems that they present, both ethically and therapeutically, will become more acute. Not only will it become progressively more difficult to decide which patients should be treated by pharmacological methods alone, but there is also the danger that such 'treatment', because of its ease of application, might degenerate into a mere attempt to make all kinds of symptoms disappear. Thus the emotional life of the patient might, to some degree, be impoverished. In the address quoted above, Pius XII also referred to 'the danger presented to the public of resorting indiscriminately to these drugs, with the sole purpose of systematically avoiding the emotional difficulties, fears and tensions which are inseparable from an active life, and one that is concerned with the everyday tasks of mankind'.

In his working paper, Ahrenfeldt drew attention to yet another aspect of the rapid onward march of pharmacological methods:

'It may also be mentioned that a new drug, procyclidine, synthesized in 1951, has proved of appreciable value in treating the mental as well as the physical symptoms of parkinsonism: it is particularly effective in the senile arteriosclerotic cases – a fact of some importance, in view of the progressively increasing number of elderly patients' (657, 658).

SOME EFFECTS OF CURRENT TRENDS
IN MENTAL HOSPITAL PRACTICE

The potential effects of current trends (1961) towards the integration of psychiatric hospitals with community mental health services have been studied by a number of writers. The WHO Expert Committee on Mental Health (155) was hopeful that, as increasing numbers of the community came into contact with patients who had been successfully treated, attitudes to mental illness based on fear and pessimism would be superseded. This Committee advocated the extension of active treatment facilities, more closely linked with the community, in the dual belief that better treatment will lead to improved acceptance of mental patients, and that increased public tolerance will be necessary before further advances in social psychiatry can be effected. The Committee thought that in places where specialist treatment is just as easily available for the mentally sick as for the physically sick, the public might be helped to the conviction that mental illness is no less susceptible to treatment and cure than physical illness.

Greenblatt et al. (167) comment on the enormous importance to the success of psychiatric treatment of the reputation of the mental hospital in the community. This may determine not only the attitudes of patients and of their relatives, but also the nature and amount of the community's contribution to the hospital programme, and the attitude of legislators who control the finances. It is pointed out that a great deal of education is still needed before the members of the community can overcome their fear of mental illness, but that hospital personnel, including patients, are potentially among the chief ambassadors of goodwill.

Undoubtedly a most complex situation is arising out of the trends, already discussed, towards diminishing numbers of patients in mental hospitals, fewer long-stay patients, and greatly increased rates of turnover and readmission. One obvious immediate effect of these changes is that the mental hospital may come to be regarded as a place that can be got into and got out of much more easily than was believed hitherto, but it may also be doubted whether patients are being retained in hospital long enough for a thorough cure to be effected. Mental hospital lore has been enriched by the wisecrack that first there was the locked door, then the open door, and now the revolving door! Another legitimate inference is that a great many patients who would previously have gone to hospital are now being kept in the community both during their first illness and during any subsequent relapses.

Thus a very different social situation is arising, bringing with it rapid changes in the factors upon which the reputation of the mental hospital depends. Perhaps community attitudes have been most immediately affected by the spread of the practice of making informal admissions to, and discharges from, mental hospitals, and by other measures leading towards the breakdown of the strict segregation of the patient from the community. In countries where these changes are occurring on a significant scale there is evidence of an increasing tendency to regard mental hospitals as places to which patients can be freely admitted and readmitted in times of need for short spells in the course of processes of rehabilitation. In a report to the United States Veterans' Administration (64) it was stated:

'Since the stigma of hospitalization in a psychiatric hospital is considerably reduced, there is easy admission to the hospital on the part of the patient, less resistance of the families on having their relatives admitted, and a considerable reduction in the difficulty of having patients returned to their homes in the community. This patient-hospital relationship, the fact that the psychiatric hospital is being considered as a hospital, is most important therapeutically. The hospital is not looked upon as a dumping ground for difficult persons in the family circle. The hospital itself, because of the easy admission policies, the vacation admissions, the emergency admissions to help families in times of stress, is considered to be a resource which backs up the family in times of need and makes for better hospital-community relationship. This does not minimize the fact that the general community and public have as much aroused feeling when incidents occur as would happen in our country. It does indicate, however, that the general relationship appears to be on a most satisfactory note.'

Parallel with the trends decreasing the remoteness of the mental hospital from the community, the development of community psychiatric services as a part of mental health facilities has been going forward. It appears to have been true, at least in some places, that experimental forms of treatment in the community, outside the walls of the mental hospital, were initiated to offset, and drew their main motive force from, the serious problem of overcrowding in psychiatric hospitals (95, 143, 145).

Cooper and Early (164) have written, with particular reference to experience in Bristol, England:

'To solve the problem of overcrowding, and to make economic use of medical and nursing staff, it is essential for mental hospitals to maintain an active discharge policy. If the mental hospital is allowed to continue to fulfil the functions of a hostel, and a geriatric and chronic-sick unit, this must deprive psychiatric patients of the care which is their right, and will serve only to discourage medical and nursing staff. Thus there is every incentive to discharge chronic mental patients from hospital whenever possible. The effect, however, of discharging psychiatric patients prematurely or without adequate provision may well be serious for the patients' relatives and for the community; moreover, such patients relapse quickly in a high proportion of cases. To pursue a deliberate policy of discharging chronic patients, without regard to the facilities existing for their resettlement, is irresponsible, and likely to discredit the whole concept of "open door" psychiatry. In short, although a large proportion of mental hospital patients may be regarded as not in need of hospital care, it is highly undesirable that they should be discharged on these grounds unless suitable alternative accommodation exists.'

This note of warning about the attendant disadvantages of current trends has been echoed by many writers; and it will illuminate this complex subject to discuss and cite some of the literature dealing with various aspects of the social difficulties and dangers involved.

Holman (151) has drawn attention to the havoc done to children who are obliged to live with a psychotic parent, and he deplores the possible consequences of the premature discharge of a parent from hospital, such as having to send the children away from home.

May (145) puts the position in a statesmanlike way as follows:

'Like other forms of treatment, community care has complications and side-effects. The patient and his relatives become impatient at slow progress . . . Initial improvement . . . may be followed by relapse, and in-patient treatment may then become imperative. The patient may increase his demands on relatives to a point where they cannot meet them, with a consequent deterioration in emotional relationships. . . . Since mental illness has many causes, its management is difficult and its correct appraisal obscure. Because of the imprecision of our knowledge, there is a real danger that we shall be subjected to external pressures in our dealings with it. Public interest has been awakened in community care, and plans bid fair to outstrip the achievement of what is both practical and proper. I do not wish to decry its advantages, but I would urge that we should strive for a more critical assessment of its aims, its indications, and its practical application.'

Ferguson (136), though fully aware of the 'dehumanizing effects of a long sojourn in the back wards of a large institution', is deeply concerned lest the remedy now being proposed fall into disrepute by over-use. He questions whether a very quick turnover of patients is necessarily virtuous and whether the patients themselves are always sufficiently consulted in the matter. He writes: 'If in the past patients were kept too long in hospital, it would be foolish to overcompensate and fall into the error of not keeping them long enough.'

Concern with the possible attendant social dangers of community treatment of psychosis is not limited to Great Britain. Leconte (476) has enumerated the large series of crimes of violence committed in France in recent years by psychiatric patients who have been prematurely discharged. (He does not include suicides and other tragedies attributable to the same cause.) His conclusion is that the people concerned were 'sacrificed to administrative expediency', and that rapid turnover only results in some of the discharged patients being subsequently readmitted to hospital on a number of occasions, each time in a slightly worse condition. Leconte takes a very serious view of the situation in France and calls for an objective investigation of relapse and recurrence in mental patients. He regards the fashion of early discharge as having harmful consequences, not only for public order and individual safety, but for mental patients themselves who, he thinks, will suffer from a deterioration in the public attitude towards patients who are recovering. Anticipating a reversal of public policy, he writes: '. . . mental patients themselves . . . when really cured, will once again see closing before them the doors which were beginning to open but which one has no right to open forcibly or surreptitiously'.

Overholser (175), referring to the United States where these tendencies have not yet become so widespread, comments: 'Instances of questionable release, although infinitesimally small in number, loom large at the moment in the public mind.' Overholser's concern is that a balance be struck between the two contending interests of protecting the community from risk and of restoring the patient to his proper life as soon as possible. He concludes: 'But on the other hand public clamour cannot be allowed to exert an inimical and retarding effect on the treatment of our patients.' It might be argued that 'public clamour', whether rational or irrational, and whether 'allowed' or not, may still prove a very considerable obstacle to progress, if planning and action are not coordinated with effective administrative and educational measures.

Sands (178) notes the alarm that a number of psychiatrists and others who have been working eagerly to accelerate hospital discharge rates are feeling about some of the results of their labours. He questions whether the community possesses the necessary techniques and facilities to justify the present trend towards early discharge, and expresses dismay at the fact that 'we are returning sick patients to homes and communities completely unsuited to deal with the problems'. Beresford (161) takes a similar view in his observation that serious overcrowding makes early discharge desirable, but that discharge may be too soon for the real interests of the patient unless there is an efficient aftercare service. He warns that aftercare is for recovered patients, to help rehabilitation and to minimize the risk of further breakdown. It is not intended to help the half-recovered person to make his adjustment outside the hospital. Beresford says that the half-recovered patient, trying to adjust to the demands of life outside the hospital, 'can often suffer or cause others to suffer far greater unhappiness than any one should really be expected to bear'.

Oliver (151), though deploring like everybody else the prison-like atmosphere of some older mental hospitals 'with so-called emphasis on lock and key and little else', feels that it is currently fashionable to disregard other considerations in the modern preoccupation with 'quick turnover of patients, low bed-occupancy rate, outpatient treatment, day hospitals, hostels, extra social workers, sheltered workshops, anything, in fact, to keep a mentally ill patient from being in an asylum, and I use the word meaningfully, and, if he is admitted, to discharge him just as soon as is humanly possible'.

The Study Group was convinced of the validity of the many warnings and criticisms that have been expressed in recent years about the current trends that have been discussed. An additional problem not mentioned so far concerns the needs of the more chronic psychotic patients who require a longer term of hospital treatment because of the slow-moving nature of their illness, and also for the sake of their families and the community. A therapeutic course for such a patient that is planned with more regard to the currently fashionable demands for quick results than to the needs of the patient himself may do more harm than good.

Another considerable danger arising from pressure for the early discharge of psychotic patients from hospital is that seriously ill patients may be sent home with their more florid symptoms masked by tranquillizing drugs. It has been noted in some countries that communication between the staff of the psychiatric hospital and the members of the family who are to take charge of the patient, and particularly the family physician, is not always, or even usually, adequate. Relatives become disturbed when a discharged patient displays symptoms, and the general practitioner, who is usually without adequate training in the management of the psychotic patient in the community, tends to return the patient to hospital. The Study Group considered that for a period of perhaps twenty years, by which time it is hoped that the majority of general practitioners will have a better understanding of the problems involved, it will be desirable for the hospital staff to take a very active part in the domiciliary treatment of newly discharged patients. As a first step in this direction there could be a wider use of psychiatric services in general hospitals.

It is apparent that the relationships between the community and the mental hospital in many countries are in a state of confusion and flux. In Great Britain, where there has been more experience of the new trends in hospital practice than in any other country, it is probably true to say that up to now there has been more clamour in the patients' interest for early discharge than opposition from an alarmed public. The Royal Commission (404) drew attention to the need to 'balance the possible benefits of treatment or training, the protection of the patient and . . . of other persons, on the one hand, against the patient's loss of liberty on the other'. On this point Ahrenfeldt has expressed the hope that such judgements be made on clinical acumen and experience rather than on administrative expediency; and he has called for an objective, statistically representative, follow-up survey of such patients (see also Kramer (110)). In Ahrenfeldt's view there are delicately balanced, reversible reactions between the hospital and the community, the profession and the community, and patients and the community; and he remarks that, although the catalysts favouring a reaction in one or the other direction are not yet sufficiently known, their influence cannot be ignored:

'We should not go faster than the available community services permit; and we should bear in mind the fact that there is frequently a lack of continuity in hospital treatment and after-care, apart from the deficiency in extramural facilities and shortage of trained personnel for these services.'

The Study Group was strongly of the opinion that a middle way should be sought through these problems. The conclusion was that the advantages of the new trends are not as overwhelming, nor their disadvantages as insignificant, as has commonly been thought up to now. As experience is gained in the increasing use of community treatment, with its emphasis on early discharge from hospital and rapid return of psychotics to the community, professional and administrative enthusiasm for the current trends may well be tempered by an awareness of the possible limitations of such methods, of the glaring deficiencies in personnel and in collaborating services, and of the inadequate state of public education for coping with the situations that may arise.

In support of the point made by Ahrenfeldt above, Ewalt, in a working paper, observed that while the goal of all this activity is to care for the patient at home whenever possible, one potential weakness is that the decision whether to leave the patient at home during the acute treatment phase tends to be based more on the tolerance of the family than on consideration of what type of handling will ultimately bring most benefit to the patient and least damage to the family.

Concerned with the same danger of the pressures of expediency, Stoller remarked in a working paper that it was not difficult to avoid many hospital admissions and readmissions by the expansion of community facilities. What was difficult was to ascertain that such a policy did not reduce meretriciously the number of mental hospital beds, by transferring psychiatric responsibilities to others (e.g. to the geriatric services), which might be less adequately equipped or not suitable at all to deal with psychiatric problems. Alternatively, these psychiatric responsibilities may be placed on families, causing children to suffer untoward effects, or saddling adult members of the family with intolerable burdens.

Other observers have expressed alarm at the way in which extramural mental health services may be improvised in an attempt to fill in gaps in the community services which deserve more considered planning in their own right. Writing of the United Kingdom, Titmuss (149) has remarked that the British tend to express aspirations in idealistic terms, but that public opinion might be confused into thinking that the aspirations had become reality merely because they had been expressed. Titmuss continued: 'If community care was to be a reality, it must start in the hospital and encompass all the social services. To scatter the mentally ill in the community without adequate provision was not a solution, even financially . . .' With reference to the ministerial statement made early in 1960, and discussed above, that it might be possible to effect a substantial reduction in the number of mental hospital beds within the next decade, Titmuss observed that this implies a remarkable degree of optimism about the rapidly rising readmission rate, and about the parts to be played by general practitioners and local health authorities. Like Stoller, he expressed concern lest the community was drifting into a situation in which care of the mentally ill was being transferred from trained staff to untrained or ill-equipped staff or no staff at all.

In spite of all the difficulties, dangers, and disadvantages discussed in the foregoing paragraphs, the strength of the modern trends towards community involvement in the treatment of psychiatric illness is impressive, and repercussions of modern thinking are being felt in other areas of the social field. A striking example is provided by the 1959 Mental Health Act in England

and Wales, which was enacted to replace all previous legislation in the field of mental disorder and mental deficiency. Among the categories of mental disturbance provided for is 'psychopathic disorder', defined as 'a persistent disorder or disability of mind (whether or not including subnormality of intelligence) which results in abnormally aggressive or seriously irresponsible conduct on the part of the patient and requires, or is susceptible to, medical treatment'. This clause has the effect of bringing psychopathic behaviour within the scope of medical treatment and has raised the significant question of a medical type of institution for the treatment of chronic criminality. If moves are made in this direction they will undoubtedly result in the provision once again of some closed or partially closed psychiatric hospitals for individuals who are there under some form of legal duress.

Thus, at a time when mental hospitals have passed through a revolutionary change resulting in the virtual disappearance of legal sanctions and locked doors, when the emphasis is on ease and informality of admission, and when the public is beginning to get used to regarding the mental hospital as a place which can be used freely for the passing problems of acute psychosis and for the orientation difficulties of old age, there has arisen a movement in the contrary direction for the application of psychiatric treatment methods to non-volitional patients under legal duress, with all the possibilities of loss of civil rights and so on that were characteristic of the old lunacy legislation. This is a paradoxical situation and represents one of the emerging problems at the end of the period under review.

THE HOSPITAL AND THE PATIENT'S FAMILY

One further specific aspect of the relationship between the psychiatric hospital and the community is the relationship between the hospital staff and the patient's family. This has been well described by Linn (243), and also by Greenblatt et al. (167) who affirm that group meetings with relatives, introduced at the Boston Psychopathic Hospital, proved of considerable value in decreasing tensions and improving the hospital–community relationship. Fleck *et al.* (165), in an initial report on a few of the many significant problems that can arise between staff and family, stated:

'In the course of our study of the family environment of schizophrenic patients . . . we have become increasingly aware of the need for constant examination of the interrelationship between the hospital staff and the families of patients. Without attention to this relationship, family attitudes toward the hospital or staff attitudes toward the family may affect the patient deleteriously or even catastrophically.'

Relevant to this point is the emphasis by Greenblatt *et al.* (167) in the United States on the importance to the hospital–community relationship of careful planning of such matters as visiting times and patterns. Barton (328) has advanced the view that the general and traditional restrictions on the visiting of patients in mental (and other) hospitals could be detrimental by decreasing contact with the outside world, and he advocates more or less unrestricted visiting of psychiatric inpatients. Barton and his colleagues (159) undertook an inquiry into the effects of unrestricted visiting in a mental hospital. A questionnaire was sent to all nursing sisters and charge nurses immediately before the introduction of unrestricted visiting, with a view to finding out their attitude to the project and the difficulties anticipated. A second questionnaire was administered six months after the introduction of the scheme, to ascertain the difficulties actually encountered at the time of its introduction, and staff reactions after six months' experience of the system. The first question-naire was also issued at a control hospital where visiting was not officially unrestricted. The results indicated that unrestricted visiting had not given rise to the difficulties expected either in frequency or in degree. The staff considered that both patients and relatives had benefited and that the disadvantages were trivial. During the six months' experiment the attitude of the nurses changed in favour of the new system. In a working paper, Ahrenfeldt observed that, however intrinsically valuable these trends may be, it is useful to recall that experiments on these lines were initiated originally in an attempt to solve problems of overcrowding and congestion in the psychiatric hospitals of various countries (95, 143, 145).

6

Non-residential Psychiatric Treatment

Figures on the trends of development of outpatients' services are not easy to obtain, but it seems that in many countries there has been a striking increase in outpatient activity since 1948. Statistics published in the United States (187) show that between 1954 and 1959 the number of outpatient clinics increased by 16 per cent, and the professional man-hours of clinic services rose by 37 per cent. Krapf and Moser (5) give data on psychiatric outpatient clinics for a number of countries:

No. of psychiatric outpatient clinics per one million population	Country
0·01–0·4	Brazil, Colombia, Pakistan, Province of Egypt (UAR), Taiwan, Thailand
0·5 –0·9	El Salvador, Peru, South Africa
1·0 –1·9	Austria, Costa Rica, Guatemala, Honduras
2·0 –4·9	Canada, Finland, Israel, Lebanon, Portugal, Switzerland
5·0 –9·9	England & Wales, Scotland, USA, USSR
10 and over	France, Ireland, Japan

They point out that these figures are not strictly comparable because of the different interpretations, in different countries, of what is a psychiatric outpatient clinic – some countries, for instance, included consultation services and outpatient treatment by psychiatric hospitals. All the countries that reported the existence of psychiatric outpatient clinics showed that the number of units had increased over the period studied (1948–60), several by 50–200 per cent. Finland now has three clinics for every one a decade ago.

Numbers of first consultations per year per 100,000 population varied from twenty-four in South Africa to 520 in Japan for the most recent year, and increases of from 14 to 200 per cent were shown, compared with ten years earlier. Numbers of total consultations per 100,000 population in the most recent year varied from 125 in South Africa to 2,030 in Japan; increases over the ten-year period range from 100 to 200 per cent. Krapf and Moser found no evidence, from their investigation, that in countries where there is a shortage of other types of provision for psychiatric care this is counteracted by widespread outpatient services.

In more recent years, considerable interest has been aroused in developing psychiatric practice around the nucleus of a *psychiatric hospital*. This was the subject of a special session of the WHO Expert Committee on Mental Health in 1957 (390, 182), on the general subject of preventive work in mental health. The Committee emphasized the view that, although it is desirable to develop outpatient clinics, to establish links between the hospital and the local public health services, and provide close liaison with other social agencies, it is a necessary prerequisite that the hospital itself should be 'open', with minimal formalities for admission and discharge; furthermore, its staff should not work exclusively within it, but should be involved in the extramural activities of the local mental health services.

MENTAL HEALTH CENTRES

There is some division of opinion as to what is the best type of organization for setting up community mental health activities. It is probably true that in most countries where these services have developed the impetus for starting has come from the psychiatric hospital, which is the only place in the community where a reservoir of trained personnel can be found. Apart from this practical advantage, however, many doubts (see 102, 150) have been expressed about the wisdom of the policy of extending psychiatric services based on the hospital. An alternative suggestion is that they should be developed around the nucleus of a mental health centre, predominantly outpatient in character, possibly with the provision of a few emergency services.

Veil (150) observes that 'it is indeed essential, in order that the hospital may provide all the services in respect of which it is irreplaceable, that it should be relieved of those tasks for which it is not suited'. In his view, it is the *dispensaire de prophylaxie mentale* that should constitute the centre of the service: it should have a welcoming atmosphere, be conveniently accessible (and open in the evening), and offer a comprehensive range of facilities (including child guidance, meetings, aftercare supervision, medical and psychological diagnostic services, social services, outpatient treatment for alcoholics, etc.).

The WHO European Conference on Mental Hygiene Practice (Helsinki, 1959) (102) listed the functions of the mental health centre as follows:

'(a) Out-patient treatment of psychiatric patients, excluding those who could be treated by general practitioners. The Committee envisaged that the general practitioner, or his equivalent, would always have to deal with a large part of the mentally ill, especially in rural areas. The relation between practitioners and the centre would be intimate, with consultation on both sides being freely available.

'(b) Aftercare of those discharged from hospital. Liaison with psychiatric hospitals should be close, and include interchange of staff.

'(c) A diagnostic service, not only for the centre's own patients, but also for patients in other services (general medicine, geriatric, etc.).

'(d) Supervision of long-term patients in their own homes.

'(e) Supervision of care in families, hostels, small homes for long-term patients, day centres, etc.

'(f) Case-finding and early detection of the mentally ill or disturbed. Collaboration with general practitioners, public health nurses, and social workers is essential for this task. More active procedures may be organized.

'(g) Social psychiatric consultations to community agencies – services for delinquents, vagabonds, alcoholics, unemployed, handicapped, etc.

'(h) Psychiatric first-aid.

'(i) Information, public education with respect to mental illness and mental health.'

This type of multipurpose mental health centre is beginning to develop, e.g. in Sweden and France (67), and has long existed in various forms in the Netherlands, sometimes in close connexion with a general health centre and general hospital, but more usually as a separate social psychiatry centre with emergency functions, preventive aims, and aftercare services, and including in its activities mental health work with children. The Soviet system, similarly, is designed to comprise all these functions and, in addition, is backed by a relatively large provision of beds, so that the same staff work with both inpatients and outpatients.

These principles were further discussed in 1960 by the WHO Expert Committee on Mental Health (391), whose report laid emphasis on the siting of the mental health centre in order to serve a defined area. Various recommendations had been put forward as to the 'ideal' size for an area, from an area comprising a population of 150,000 (as in Paris) to one comprising 500,000 (as in Moscow). In the United Kingdom, an area contains, on average, a population of some 300,000. The size of the area must obviously depend upon local administrative considerations, and upon whether it is located in a densely populated urban region or a more sparsely populated rural district. An earlier (1953) WHO Expert Committee on Mental Health (195) had observed:

'At first sight, it may seem that to establish a psychiatric out-patient service as soon as the need for emergency custodial care is met, is an unrealistic way in which to employ the staff of the community mental hospital. But upon reflection it will be evident that out-patient work is in effect the antenna of the community mental hospital, and that from the clinical experience of this service may be derived the most reliable indicators of the direction in which the hospital should develop if it is to meet the needs of the community it serves.'

AMBULATORY AND DISTRICT
MENTAL HEALTH SERVICES

Questions of density of population and transport facilities limit the usefulness of the static outpatient clinic or mental health centre. There are a few examples in various countries of mobile mental health services in rural districts, in the form of teams that visit areas regularly according to a published timetable. The most interesting use of this method has been made in the prairie provinces of Canada, e.g. Saskatchewan. Fifteen years ago there were mental health clinics only in the two largest towns, with mobile or part-time clinics visiting three small centres each month. Now these three centres and one other have full-time clinics, and part-time clinics have been opened up in fifteen centres which had no services at all a decade or so ago. In Alberta there are forty part-time clinics on a travelling basis.

Emergency services operate in a number of cities, of which a notable example is the Amsterdam service pioneered by Querido. In Great Britain and Northern Ireland, the National Health Service operates a domiciliary psychiatric consultation service, which is available anywhere in the country.

Some recent developments in community action have a similar function to that of ambulatory mental health services, for example, the self-help organizations of patients that have sprung up in many parts of the world in relation to alcoholism, neurosis, drug addiction – Alcoholics Anonymous, among others. There are also useful parent organizations for the support of mentally defective children in a number of countries. More recently, an attempt has been made to combat suicide in cases of acute social crisis by immediate social aid, pioneered by the Samaritans in various countries. In some countries, for example UAR Province of Egypt, and Brazil, rural health centres are being equipped for psychiatric consultation, and such centres exist in more urban areas in Mexico and Panama.

COMMUNITY EXTENSION OF HOSPITAL TREATMENT

The general movement towards the liberalization of mental hospital treatment that has included informal admission, open-door wards, wider outpatient services, and the like, has also extended to the provision in certain places of part-time hospital treatment in various forms.

The impetus for this extension appears to have come from the development of what were described by Curle and Trist (541) as 'transitional communities' concerned with 'social reconnection'. The most interesting early examples of these transitional communities were the Civil Resettlement Units of the British Army (131) for the rehabilitation of repatriated prisoners from World War II. The basic idea was that the patients under treatment should become accustomed to civil life and work, while still remaining under the direction of the psychiatric treatment units.

In mental health rehabilitation work in civil life, the role of the rehabilitation centre – valuable though this has been in certain instances, e.g. the Roffey Park Industrial Rehabilitation Centre at Horsham, England – has not been as large as that of part-time hospital care. Of the latter type of provision, the most widespread example has been the day hospital, which was introduced independently in 1946 by Cameron (200) in Montreal and Bierer (197) in London, and has subsequently been established in many places. There is evidence of some day-hospital development in the Soviet Union before 1946. The idea of the day hospital is that patients, who are sleeping and spending some of their leisure time in their own homes, should go to it daily, for a period roughly equivalent to working or office hours, and there receive individual and group psychiatric treatment.

A counterpart that is administratively logical is the night hospital, and in this case the patients undergo specialized psychiatric treatment in the hospital in the evenings, and sleep there, while working during the day locally in the community. In some places the attempt has been made to use the same set of premises for the two sets of patients, on a day- and a night-hospital basis respectively; but the administrative complications involved perhaps negate much of the value of the increase in the treatment potential of a single unit.

The provision of day hospitals has spread quite widely in a number of parts of the world, though figures are incomplete. In Krapf and Moser's survey (5), seventy-six day hospitals and fifty-three night hospitals are reported in the United States. The night hospital has not been so widely developed, but estimates of this type of provision would have to take account of the fact that it has been the custom, in a great number of mental hospitals, for certain patients to work in the community and to return to the hospital at night, and no figures are available about the extent of these practices. A particularly interesting experimental day hospital was successfully established in 1954 in Western Nigeria, and the method used there is advocated as being especially suitable for countries with a great shortage of personnel. Lambo (73) writes:

'Where family units are so close and interpersonal relations are so important, experience has shown that patients should be treated in as natural an environment as possible. . . . At the outset of this experimental day hospital, the *bales* (the village heads) of the four big villages were interviewed, and all plans were explained to them and their co-operation was sought. . . . Patients are accompanied by their relatives, usually either mother, sister, brother, or aunt, and most of them come from distant areas. A nurse is always on duty in the village at night to cope with the minor nursing exigencies (insomnia, head-aches, etc.) and to send for help in matters of urgency. . . . A guide is also provided by the hospital to look after the relatives of patients from distant areas.'

There is a good deal of difference of opinion about the value of these kinds of development, but Bierer (197) has claimed that a 'mental health service centred round the comprehensive day hospital, with a night hospital, therapeutic community hostel, therapeutic social clubs, self-governed workshops, and a small community service, could fulfil most future needs'.

Other types of transitional community have been traditional in psychiatric practice in many parts of the world. These include working villages, of which the best known is Gheel in Belgium, which has been operating for several hundred years; and halfway houses, sheltered workshops, and so on. It is hard to estimate the growth in these facilities that has occurred since 1948, but it appears that there have been rapid recent developments in Western Europe and North America of the specialized industrial unit that can occupy psychiatric patients gainfully under protected conditions and, if required, on a long-term basis. A good example of this is the Cheadle Royal Hospital in Cheshire, England, where chronic psychiatric patients living either in the hospital or in the local community are employed on factory work.

An introduction of more industrial types of work is causing considerable change in the older-established ideas of occupational therapy. Traditionally, occupational therapy both in general and in psychiatric hospitals has, as the name suggests, been based on the provision of suitable activities to occupy patients' minds and hands while they are in bed, and during early convalescence. The current trends towards work-oriented occupational therapy appear to be spreading around the world. Krapf and Moser (5) report an enormous increase in the facilities offered in many countries, and an expansion of training programmes for occupational therapists. In Western Europe, North America, and other countries such as Japan and Israel, every mental hospital has its occupational therapy department staffed by trained therapists. There is now, however, a developing body of opinion that advocates a change of emphasis in relation to occupational therapy over and above the trend to give patients productive work to do rather than mere 'occupation'. More and more nurses are being involved in responsibility for patients' programmes of daily work or occupation. It is considered logical that the nurses who look after the patients during the rest of the day should be with them during their work periods, so that a more complete integration of the various aspects of mental hospital life may be achieved.

In some countries the work programme of patients is tending to develop outside the psychiatric hospital proper. Israel has pioneered the provision of 'work villages' with a more active programme of rehabilitation by work than has usually been the case in traditional settlements. In many other countries a considerable number of psychiatric patients are currently engaged in direct work of an industrial or commercial type within the hospital, or are found productive employment in the local community as part of the therapeutic programme.

Among halfway houses there are apparently no definite new trends, and those that do exist appear to vary greatly in their orientation in different countries. The more traditional attitude has been to provide a sheltered environment in which patients can live a trouble-free existence. The movement towards converting these places into more actively rehabilitating types of community, with a short-term objective of returning the patients to life outside, has not, as far as we can make out, assumed impressive proportions in any country.

The organization of these various forms of community treatment, aftercare, and rehabilitation for those who have been mentally ill is a complex matter, which varies very much according to the structure of the local community, the population density, and the existing social tradition of organization for the health and welfare services. Conditions in different countries are so diverse that no general trends can be seen. It is worth mentioning that, in the United Kingdom, where the introduction of the National Health Service in 1948 placed mental treatment and rehabilitation on the same basis as all other forms of medical service, the administrative solution adopted has been to make hospital treatment the responsibility of regional boards specially set up for this purpose, and all aftercare and rehabilitation measures following the patient's discharge from hospital the responsibility of the local health authorities. This arrangement has been severely criticized in various circles on the grounds that it drives an artificial wedge between two parts of the therapeutic process, and in many areas attempts are being made to resolve this weakness by the joint use of professional personnel by the separate authorities, and by other cooperative devices.

It is widely agreed in the United Kingdom that the present system has a number of major administrative shortcomings. In their study of the arrangements for rehabilitation in the Bristol area, Cooper and Early (164) comment:

'There is no clearly defined point at which the care of a chronic mental patient should be transferred from hospital staff to local authority. We believe that in the long run only joint schemes, which have in addition the cooperation and goodwill of local industry as well as of the major voluntary organizations, can successfully deal with the problem. If aftercare accommodation is to be provided by the local authority, hospital psychiatrists and social workers who are already familiar with the patients should participate in their supervision; similarly, hospital nursing staff should play a part in the care of those of their former patients who go to training workshops. . . .

'The pattern of the mental hospital is changing, and must continue to change. To obtain current information on the needs of mental patients in Bristol, and in particular on the need for aftercare facilities, a survey was made of the mental hospital population. The present situation was thought to be of particular interest in view of the development of industrial therapy and the increase in patients' earning power.

'The results suggest that little more than half the population require psychiatric hospital treatment; one-third are over the age of 65; one-third are suitable for after-care accommodation of one type or another, and of this group a high proportion are potentially self-supporting.

'There is urgent need for the provision of aftercare

accommodation, but this must be regarded as a step on the road to complete resettlement.'

PSYCHIATRIC TREATMENT AND THE GENERAL HOSPITAL
A trend that has gained ground rapidly in the last few years has been towards the comprehensive care of all the sick in a single institution. The practice of psychiatry in general hospitals has been described by Bennet *et al.* in the United States (237, 238). There appear to be two main approaches: to combine all hospital functions under one roof, as advocated by Brook and Stafford-Clark (239); and, perhaps more commonly, to establish a psychiatric unit in the grounds of a general hospital or contiguous to it. In the Manchester Hospital Region of the United Kingdom it has become the policy to transfer psychiatric hospital patients, as opportunity offers, to small psychiatric units in the grounds of general hospitals (242, 247). In Bolton and Oldham, Lancashire, United Kingdom (94, 96), district psychiatric services have been organized on this principle. A Danish Commission to advise on the State Mental Health Service recommended that future psychiatric hospitals should be built in close connexion with general hospitals, and that their size should not exceed 350 beds (84).

Further examples of these trends are to be found in various other parts of the world: e.g. in South Africa (245); in Queensland, Australia (246), where small annexes for senile mental patients have been developed, or planned, in general hospitals; and in the (US) Virgin Islands (9), where all the psychiatric in-patients are cared for in a wing of the general hospital, and move around as freely as ambulant patients in any other ward.

The WHO seminar on mental health in Africa, 1958 (91), noted that, in Africa, mental illness is often associated with or caused by physical factors, and recommended the use of numerous small centres combined with general hospital services. It is interesting that the general hospital at Usumbura (Ruanda Urundi) has been treating its psychiatric cases in open wards for several years.

Krapf and Moser (5) estimated the number of beds in psychiatric wards in general hospitals in several countries. In most of these countries the number had increased by 50 to 130 per cent over the period of their survey.

No. of beds per 100,000 population	Country
1–4	Austria, Israel, New Zealand, Peru, Portugal
5–9	Canada, USA, Yugoslavia
10–14	Honduras
15–19	Japan, Sweden, UK

In a working paper, Ewalt drew attention to the study made by the US Joint Commission on Mental Illness and Health (389) of ways in which new programmes could be instituted without giving rise to major social stress, and without requiring changes in legislation or involving large increases in money costs.

There has been an increase of 27 per cent, in a four-year period, in the use of general hospital facilities for the care of mental patients in the state of New York. For example, during 1958, 6,800 hospitals in the United States admitted 23 million patients and gave 143 million days of hospital care. Of the mental patients in this total of admissions, 257,000 were admitted to general hospitals and 210,000 to mental hospitals. One significant result of this striking trend is that the creation of small psychiatric units in general hospitals is encouraging psychiatrists to move out from the larger urban areas, because they can now earn a living in smaller places. This dispersal of psychiatric skill is also to the advantage of family physicians in the smaller centres. A similar trend is current in the United Kingdom, and has been evident for some time, we understand, in the Soviet Union. A problem in these countries appears to be not so much the encouragement of such practices as their management.

In the United Kingdom the long-term policy is to encourage the setting up, in general hospitals, of psychiatric units, comprising a minimum of a hundred beds, and capable of offering the full range of services that are available in the best mental hospitals today. It is hoped that with the achievement of this policy the other departments of the general hospital will benefit greatly from the presence of the psychiatric unit, not least from the demonstration of how to look after a patient throughout the twenty-four hours of the day – the whole patient, and not only his illness.

The most recent recommendation in the United States, by the Joint Commission on Mental Illness and Health (389), follows closely similar lines:

'*General hospital psychiatric units:* No community general hospital should be regarded as rendering a complete service unless it accepts mental patients for short-term hospitalization and therefore provides a psychiatric unit or psychiatric beds. Every community general hospital of 100 or more beds should make this provision. A hospital with such facilities should be regarded as an integral part of a total system of mental patient services in its region. It is the consensus of the Mental Health Study that definitive care for patients with major illness should be given if possible, or for as long as possible, in a psychiatric unit of a general hospital and then, on a longer term basis, in a specialized mental hospital organized as an intensive psychiatric treatment centre.'

These tendencies to place the treatment of psychiatric patients in general hospitals are not without critics. The WHO Expert Committee (195) in its third report dissented from the widely expressed view that psychiatric wards in general hospitals are necessarily or invariably the most desirable form of provision for psychiatric care, and its dissent is echoed by Repond (176). The place of inpatient psychiatry in the general hospital has recently been the subject of searching and critical appraisal, for example, in the United Kingdom (169, 240, 248). As stated in the *Lancet* (185):

'The proposition that most psychiatric treatment will shortly move from mental to general hospitals has provoked surprisingly little contention. What criticism there has been of this phase of hospital replanning has not been very cogent, and particular attention will therefore be paid to a careful and comprehensive account of *Mental Hospitals at Work* by Dr Kathleen Jones and Prof. Roy Sidebotham (169). . . . The prime argument is whether or not psychiatric units can work well in general hospitals,'

and these authors believe that they are unsuitable for most patients: 'The treatment of mental illness is more exacting in many ways than that of physical illness, and a psychiatric unit designed on the lines of general medical and surgical wards would be a disaster.' However, the *Lancet* concludes:

'The progress achieved in mental-hospital psychiatry has made it possible for these hospitals to extend their activities into the general hospitals. The continuance of this trend can benefit the psychiatrists, their patients, and those of their medical and surgical colleagues who have worked too long in isolation from the emotions and personalities of their patients.'

There has been considerable discussion of this question also in the state of Victoria, Australia, where psychiatric units in general hospitals have been strongly advocated. However, it was reported that there is a body of opinion there that holds that, since psychiatric patients are ambulatory and their rehabilitation requires facilities for both work and recreational programmes, it is a seriously mistaken policy to attempt to apply to psychiatric units either the staff–patient attitudes or the physical structure of the general hospital. Many people have concluded that the time is not yet ripe for the full integration of modern psychiatric concepts with general medical practice; that, for the time being, it may be advisable to have psychiatric units adjacent to, and serving, general hospitals, and to work, at the same time, towards the permeation of the general hospital atmosphere with psychiatric concepts of handling patients. This last point is especially relevant in view of the fact that general hospitals have always had a goodly percentage of cases that are essentially psychiatric, though not always consciously recognized as such.

The Study Group devoted a good deal of discussion to the complex issues involved in expanding psychiatric treatment within the general hospital. It was emphasized by a psychiatrist that general hospitals offer different facilities from those of mental hospitals, and deal for the most part with aspects of mental illness that are not primarily the responsibility of the mental hospital services. The services provided at present by the general hospitals are especially useful for the treatment of neurosis and psychosomatic disorders, for the teaching of undergraduates, and for the infiltration of medical and surgical specialities. In addition, the more highly specialized psychiatric services are extending into a much broader field of social and educational action than that of traditional medicine. Although it may be felt that these extensions are very properly and immediately the concern of medical science and practice, it cannot be claimed that they are within the present frame of general medicine.

The Study Group considered the readiness of general hospitals to take over responsibility for the treatment of acute psychosis. In recent years the whole philosophy of psychiatric therapy has moved away from bed-centred therapeutics and rest into the social sphere of interpersonal relationships. There is necessarily a considerable time lag between the introduction of new techniques in medicine and the emergence into influential positions of a new generation of doctors who are identified with the new attitudes. Therefore a vast and urgent programme of medical re-education will have to be undertaken concurrently with, or preferably in advance of, the transfer of psychiatric hospital patients to general hospitals. It will not be enough to import existing mental hospital staffs together with their patients into general hospitals, because the whole philosophy of mental hospital treatment will probably prove severely disturbing to the traditional atmosphere of a general medical and surgical hospital.

It is legitimate to hope that the orientation of psychiatric treatment will permeate the general hospital and foment there the mental hospital's revolutionary change of attitude towards seeing the patient as a human being and as a member of the community. But it cannot be expected that such a transition will work smoothly, or invariably beneficially, for the psychiatric patient.

7
Some Mental Health Problems in Society

The tremendous expansion in recent years of psychiatric services in various forms – including the development of the therapeutic atmosphere of the psychiatric hospital, the extension of outpatient services, the provision of day and night hospitals and so on, together with the introduction of successful physical and psychopharmacological techniques – has given a rapidly growing impetus to the experimental use of community services. Hospital staffs working extramurally have been responsible for the attempts made in this area in many countries, but it appears that nowhere are there sufficient staff and adequate facilities to makes these services really effective. A primary need, almost everywhere, is to involve the other services in the community, and the citizens generally, in the work of early recognition of psychiatric disorder and of reintegration of the patient into the community.

Much of the work involving the community must necessarily stem from the psychiatric hospital itself because, in most communities, this is the only centre where the essential skills and experience are concentrated.

The evolutionary trends of the relationship between psychiatric hospital and community in Western Europe and North America, and those now reflected in the planning and development of mental health services in various other parts of the world, have been well summarized by Macmillan (143). This author, advocating a comprehensive community service to treat all types of mental illness (including the chronic psychoses) at all stages, writes:

'This means that the mental hospital must take an active part in the scheme and is the most practical way of using our existing resources. It also means that we must alter our attitude to the chronic patients, and establish a personal relationship with them. . . . The function of the hospital is altered and modified, so that it becomes only one part, but an essential part, of the service. The resources and energies which would otherwise be spent providing long-term residential accommodation for patients can be diverted to domiciliary and community activities. . . . The patient retains his social and economic independence, and the mental hospital, like the general hospital, offers him specialized inpatient treatment when the resources of the home, and the domiciliary and community services, become temporarily unable to cope with his illness.

'For a comprehensive scheme to be successful, the following conditions are essential: integration of the hospital service with the local health authority; removal of barriers isolating the hospital from the community; an internal psychotherapeutic atmosphere in the hospital; and an enlightened and informed public opinion in the community. . . .

'To sum up, community treatment not only makes possible continuity of care for all forms of psychiatric illness, but by its beneficial influence on public opinion persuades patients and their relatives to come spontaneously to the mental health department for help and advice, and to accept the mental hospital, like the general hospital, as a place where the patient goes to speed his rehabilitation.

'Evaluation of the benefit offered to the psychiatric patient by community treatment must await scientific appraisal, but its advantages are already sufficiently clear to justify a critical attitude towards rigid measures of long-term hospital treatment. The possible methods of providing this treatment should be given a practical trial, and the results of these experimental schemes studied carefully, so that we may, in due course, judge which is best for the patient.'

Essential prerequisities of effective community treatment are the early recognition of those disorders that are suitable for hospital treatment, and the capacity to undertake suitable prophylactic action in the community. In a number of places, networks of prophylaxis have been set up, which successfully combine the functions of rehabilitation and reintegration of the patient with the task of making the community more aware of the realities of psychiatric disorders and more able to take effective early action. An example of what can be achieved is provided by the state of Victoria, Australia, where regional psychiatric services have been developing through the use of the community network of advisory services, social therapeutic clubs, day centres for the mentally retarded, hostels, outpatient clinics, day hospitals, sheltered workshops, early treatment centres, and short-stay and long-stay rehabilitation hospitals. The mental health services are called upon to provide specialized care in all the ramifications of these various activities.

There is less that can be written cross-culturally about community measures to secure early consultation and therefore early recognition of psychiatric disorders. This is partly due to the lack of comparable terminology in various countries. It has been emphasized in a number of countries where there have been projects to institute what have sometimes been described as 'pre-treatment services' that it is extremely important to ensure that facilities for consultation do not outrun the treatment and the prophylactic measures that are available. Should this happen, the legacy of anxiety in the community may be considerable.

In a number of countries two major streams of development are going on side by side: (i) the provision of *domiciliary* advisory and therapeutic services; (ii) the provision of *emergency* services (or 'psychiatric first aid') on a twenty-four-hour basis. The classic example is that of the Amsterdam Municipal Psychiatric Services, which are now a well-established part of the organization built up by Querido (95, 98, 99) and his colleagues over a number of years. These services are designed not only to meet local needs, but more especially to relieve the serious pressure of increasing demands made on limited inpatient accommodation.

Emergency psychiatric clinics have been established in a number of places, e.g. at the Maudsley Hospital, London (203), and at the Bronx Mental Hospital, New York (93). The latter has as its objective the reduction of barriers between patient and psychiatrist, by facilitating consultation when it is most needed.

In addition, emergency services have been started in a number of places in respect of specific problems referred to above, notably alcoholism and drug addiction. More recently established, and with less general application so far, are emergency services to deal with acute psychological and social distress which is leading towards suicide. In one London example the service started with a telephone network, through which the suicidal individual was able to telephone a number, and was given the name of a person near his home to contact; the respondents in the scheme having being mobilized to be on call. This initiative has evolved in a number of other centres in various parts of the world into the provision of a twenty-four-hour clinical and social service – under the name of 'Samaritans'.

In a working paper, Ahrenfeldt commented:

'Domiciliary treatment has also been used increasingly, for example, in the United Kingdom, as part of certain well-organized community psychiatric services. It has been employed extensively in the Worthing Experiment (92) and in Nottingham (143, 172), and also to some extent in the Bolton (96) and Oldham (94) district psychiatric services. Macmillan (143) states: "One definite advantage of community treatment is that by means of domiciliary visits psychiatric illness is treated at an even earlier stage than is possible with the out-patient clinic. In an integrated mental health service the home and health visitors recognize psychiatric situations before serious symptoms have developed. Potential stages of a serious breakdown can be treated, and prophylactic measures started in a way which is impossible without a community service."

'Domiciliary visits have, however, not in general yet assumed large proportions, as they are necessarily time-consuming, and require a well-organized community mental health service, with a sufficient number of trained professional personnel for this particular purpose.

'As recently suggested by the WHO Expert Committee (313), domiciliary services have in fact been found of particular value in the care and treatment of elderly psychiatric patients in the home, thus, in many cases, preventing deterioration, and need for hospitalization, and the breaking up of the family (382).'

FOSTER FAMILY CARE

It is perhaps paradoxical that whereas the placing of the main burden of psychiatric care on the natural families of patients is a recent emphasis, the employment of foster families for care is old established. It does not appear that there have been any significant changes in the use of foster care since 1948. As far as we have been able to discover, in no country have foster homes so far played a large part, numerically, in the care of the mentally ill, but they make a valuable contribution in some countries to the care of children, and especially of mental defectives. Thus Krapf and Moser (5) report that Austria has some 3,000 foster-home places; Finland, 900; Scotland, 292 for mentally ill patients and 2,533 for mental defectives under statutory supervision in the community; and in the United States the number of patients in family care from public mental hospitals has increased, from less than 5,000 in 1951 to 12,500 in 1960. In England and Wales the placement of mentally ill patients in foster homes has probably been on a larger scale than in any of the countries mentioned, but exact figures are not available. Foster-home care has certainly been important there in respect of mental defectives, of whom there are some 80,000 living in the community under some form of supervision, including supervision in their own families, as compared with approximately 50,000 in residential institutions.[1]

[1] These were the figures made available to the Study Group. It is known that, in most countries of Europe and in many countries elsewhere, there are patients under foster-home care. Among European countries, in addition to those already mentioned, this method of care has been most employed in France, Belgium, and the Netherlands. The Scandinavian countries all have large numbers of mental defectives under foster-home care.

MENTAL HEALTH PROBLEMS
OF CHILDREN AND ADOLESCENTS

On the whole, progress made in the postwar period in psychiatric work with children and adolescents has been disappointing. The concept of child guidance as a sphere of interdisciplinary cooperation, as associated with the name of Healey in Chicago in the first decade of this century, has developed to a significant extent in comparatively few countries and has not made the general impact in the last fifty years that at one time looked likely. There appear to be many reasons for this – a major one being that child guidance, with its network of interdisciplinary cooperation, requires for successful operation a complex and sophisticated level of organization of the social welfare services in the community. A second reason for slow and patchy progress is that child psychiatry, of all branches of psychiatry, is the most involved in patterns of family life and the functioning of the culture generally. It is therefore the least exportable across cultural boundaries. In no respect has this complication of cultural differences been felt more strongly than in the evolution of a theoretical basis for clinical practice. As discussed in Chapter 3, even within a single culture there is at present little agreement on principles of psychopathology and aetiology, a situation with serious consequent difficulties in professional training. A further feature hampering growth has been the fact that in most countries the majority of professional people have entered the field of child psychiatry from a basis of training in the principles of adult psychiatry, so that the specific psychiatric problems of children have nowhere received the attention that they need, free from preconceptions from other fields of study.

The difficulties that psychiatrists have experienced, in most of the interested countries, in attempting to develop a genuine science of child psychiatry are not, of course, the only reason for the continued weakness of this subject. The collaborating professions of psychology and social work have also had to contend with difficulties deriving from past professional orientation. In most countries psychologists have approached the problems of child guidance from a previous experience of education, and social workers from general social welfare work, and in both cases their specific techniques for child guidance have been slow in evolving. It may be noted here that it has been not uncommonly found in newly developing branches of medicine, e.g. paediatrics, that progress has been slow until positions of influence have been attained by a strong body of professional people born and bred in the new discipline, as it were, and able to view its problems from within and not from the standpoint of someone trained in another discipline and applying this previous experience to a new set of factors. This new generation is only beginning to emerge in a few countries, but there is now a growing volume of literature dealing with various aspects of child guidance problems: e.g. from the practical aspect (18); from the preventive aspect (418); and from the point of view of a search for a more specific nosology and general theoretical background (278).

Although the progress in mental health work among children has been disappointingly slow in most countries, yet it is true in principle that in every country where welfare work with children is attempted there is some recognition of the need to do more than deal merely with problems of mental deficiency and gross pathology. In most of the countries of Europe and North America there are more or less comprehensive systems of psychological and social services for children, in line with modern mental health principles, offering counselling and guidance in connexion with child welfare (well-baby) clinics, and comparable facilities in respect of children with educational and behavioural difficulties, and children who are delinquent or suffering severe mental retardation or disorder. Out of a wide field of modern developments in provisions for children with educational and behavioural difficulties at home and in school, we have space to mention only one or two.

In the United States there has been a general expansion of psychological counselling services integrated with the school system and also relating closely to parents through parent-teacher cooperation. We would draw attention in particular to the use of school counsellors who are members of school staffs and specialized in understanding the psychological difficulties of children.

In Great Britain the implementation of the Education Act of 1944, which included provisions for children with psychological problems no less than for those with physical handicaps, has resulted in a widespread move towards the integration of special education facilities for so-called maladjusted children, including arrangements for special home teaching, day special schools and classes, residential schools where psychological treatment is available, and the aftercare of maladjusted children (288).

It has not proved possible to gain any idea of the extent of child guidance clinics and similar social provisions in the various countries, partly because of the absence of comparable records, but perhaps more because of the wide variations in the interpretation of these terms from country to country. Thus in some countries child guidance clinics are provided as part of the educational system and the problems are approached from an educational angle; elsewhere, and often in the same countries, other clinics are established under general hospital auspices, and still others are conducted by mental hospitals. Many clinics and centres are intended for the parents rather than for the children concerned, and there is a movement for the establishment of family guidance centres, which are, again, variously interpreted in different parts of the world.

No country that we know of reports an adequate provision of facilities for the problems of children, but it seems to be a widespread experience that the greater the attempt to provide help with these problems, the more the facilities are used and the greater the realization of the need for them. Some countries report a big increase in their activities in these fields in the post-war period.

Some specific disorders of children have recently attracted more attention. Apart from problems of retardation, which are considered below, the areas in which most interest has been expressed are those of the more severe behaviour disorders, ranging from delinquency and psychopathic behaviour on the one hand to child psychosis on the other. Everywhere there is a severe shortage of suitable accommodation for seriously disturbed and psychotic children. It is, perhaps, the case that nobody knows what is the best sort of accommodation and the most appropriate form of treatment for these children. The whole question of requirements and of the need for research into the psychiatric inpatient treatment of children was the subject of a conference in Washington, D.C., in 1956 (281), and an experimental unit to study this problem was established in England in 1954 (361). The figures that are available about existing accommodation are impressive in their inadequacy. For example, in the United Kingdom there are ten units, ranging from twenty to sixty beds each, for severely disturbed and psychotic children, and two units (thirty-four and fifty-four beds) for adolescents. This is to serve a child population of approximately 13 million. We have been informed of the existence but not of the size of approximately thirty-five residential treatment centres for disturbed children in the United States that are catering for a population at risk of the order of 45 million. It is probably true of all countries where residential treatment facilities are provided for severely disturbed children that most of the units offer a mental hospital type of care. Facilities for enabling the rehabilitation of children who have been disturbed and their return into the general stream of education are usually very poor indeed.

CHILDREN IN HOSPITAL

One outstanding recent development that is still restricted to only a few countries has been a virtual revolution in attitude towards the care of young children in hospital. Already, some fifteen years ago, Bowlby (407) in his study of maternal deprivation in children, with the support of many experienced workers in this field, specifically emphasized the need for continuity of maternal care in the case of children who were separated from their mothers and family environment, whether because of admission to a paediatric hospital, convalescent home, or specialized psychiatric unit or because of the mother's temporary or permanent removal from the home. The movement that Bowlby has been instrumental in starting in the United Kingdom, where it has gained a firm hold, has spread to a number of countries in the British Commonwealth and in Europe and, to a less extent, to the United States. There is an increasing number of reports of new attitudes to children in hospital spreading to other continents, too.

In principle, it is now accepted, in places where this radical change of attitude has been adopted, that it is better both for the children and for the hospital for the former to remain in frequent and constant touch with their parents throughout their stay in hospital; that it is better for hospital efficiency for parents to have relatively free access to their children than for restrictions to be placed on visiting on the grounds of interrupting the nursing staff or for what is now recognized to be the specious reason of the danger of cross-infection. Thus children's hospitals in the United Kingdom encourage, or it might be said expect, parents to arrange for their young children to be visited by someone close to the child for periods of at least one hour daily, and to make additional visits as required by the needs of the individual child. In the case of very young children, where the mother's other family commitments permit and, of more practical importance, where accommodation is available, the mother may be admitted too, and share in the hospital care of her baby. These changes, and the new attitude of hospital staff members towards the emotional relationships of children which the changes imply, are still strongly resisted in many parts of the world, but it has been a striking experience in the countries where they have been adopted that there is no public movement to return to the old ways. Indeed, at the time of going to press we have received news of no authenticated instance of a children's hospital going back to the discouragement of visiting – on the contrary, there are signs in a number of countries of the extension of the principle of unrestricted visiting to many types of hospital, general, maternity, children's, and psychiatric.

STUDENT MENTAL HEALTH SERVICES

Services for students in higher education fall into the borderland between the services for children and adolescents on the one hand and for adults on the other, and until recently they have been relatively neglected in most countries. There has been a recent great increase in interest in student mental hygiene, and a large number of universities all over the world are now providing some form of mental health counselling or psychiatric treatment services as part of the general medical care of students. Two useful conferences have been held on the subject – one at Princeton, New Jersey, in 1956 (453, 454); the other at Morat, Switzerland, in 1961, a European Conference of Experts on Student Mental Health, under the auspices of the World University Service. The reader is referred to the reports of these conferences for further discussion of this subject.

MENTAL DEFICIENCY

The postwar period has seen a considerable rebirth of concern with mental deficiency in children and adults in many countries. The main advances are in the education of retarded children, in social care, and in prophylactic measures in respect of organic causes of deficiency.

International interest in this subject has been reflected in a meeting of the WHO Expert Committee devoted to the mentally subnormal child in 1953 (366), a WHO European Region Seminar in 1957 (367), a WFMH report in 1959 (11), and an international conference on the scientific aspects of mental deficiency in London in 1960. There have been a great number of other meetings and small conferences. The practical problems concerning diagnosis, treatment, education, and the vocational and social rehabilitation of mentally defective children and adults have been reviewed in America, Great Britain, and other countries (362, 364).

On the side of education a significant development has occurred in Great Britain in the integration of special schools for mentally defective (now termed subnormal) children in the state education system at a lower level of educational potential than hitherto provided for, and in the provision of special training centres by local health authorities for imbecile (now termed severely subnormal) children deemed to be incapable of profiting from more formal schooling. It is now the statutory duty of local government in Great Britain to provide some suitable form of educational and training facilities for all retarded children capable of response. Similar developments are taking place in the United States where the problems of local organization are more complex owing to the federal structure, and also in a number of other countries.

On the side of social care and increasingly, too, of education, the most useful development in many countries has been the formation of associations by the parents of mentally handicapped children. These, in some places, because of their drive and involvement, have been able to do more than the authorities could do to alert the community to the needs of handicapped children and to obtain special provisions for them. This parent movement is developing alongside similar parent movements for other classes of handicapped child, e.g. children suffering from the after-effects of poliomyelitis, from brain damage, and so on. A major step forward in the social care of mentally defective children was made in the United Kingdom as a result of the Mental Health Act of 1959, which removed the certification procedure from mental deficiency provisions (now termed mental subnormality). Thus the admission of mental defectives to hospital in the United Kingdom, when necessary, is no longer under certificate but purely informal, like any other hospital admission, and, in the case of children, requires only parental consent. Retention of patients in hospital against the parents' will has similarly been done away with, except for certain provisions in case of emergency, or of danger to the child or community.

In all countries it appears that the days of the big closed mental deficiency colony are over, and, as far as information is available, few are now being constructed. In countries where such places have not been built, active consideration is being given to other forms of treatment; and in some countries where colonies exist, measures are being pursued to liberalize the atmosphere and, in principle, to reduce their size and the sense of remoteness from the community that they may experience.

In place of the big institution, new forms of part-institution/ part-home care are being explored, e.g. part-time stay in institutions, daily attendance at industrial-type workshops, cottage-style homes, daily work under contract with individual employers or in sheltered employment outside the institution while sleeping in a hostel, and so on. It is recognized that there will continue to be a need for the custodial type of institution for those individuals who, because of physical and mental difficulties, or lack of possibility of care in their family, are best off in a protected hospital-type atmosphere where their needs can be ministered to effectively and economically. For such people much greater possibilities of sheltered employment within the institution are now being explored, and there are many instances on record where quite low-grade imbeciles are being successfully employed on specially designed industrial processes.

In addition to their custodial role, institutions in many countries are now undertaking training schemes for young defectives, with the objective of helping them to re-enter normal community life and be at least partly self-supporting. Such training programmes are more and more including instruction in ordinary daily living: simple items of social behaviour, such as shopping, how to order a meal in a restaurant, make a telephone call, and so on. In order to fulfil its role properly, a training institution needs to have very close links with the community it serves, and there should be a free interchange of personnel and patients between hospital and community.

Perhaps the growing edge of the social care of mental defectives in many countries is the improvement of measures for the care of handicapped children who are living in their own homes or, in cases of necessity, in foster homes under family conditions. Thus, as remarked above, in England and Wales some 80,000 mental defectives are living in the community under the supervision of local health authorities. This figure represents about one in six hundred of the total population.

As stated elsewhere, the social care of mental defectives in the community is not new; in fact, in some instances, as at Gheel, it has been going on since the Middle Ages. What is new in the countries where these socialization services are evolving is a wider realization of both the limitations and the possibilities of subnormals living in the community. In the United Kingdom, for example, an enormous fillip has been given to this work by experience gained during World War II, when mental defectives who had been enlisted in the army were found to be causing a disproportionate amount of trouble in their units. The difficulties virtually disappeared when the defectives were remustered in special Pioneer Corps units, not armed with offensive weapons, but employed on road-building and other constructional duties, or on docks and railways, at a level of complexity of life that was within their grasp. This experience, together with other wartime measures such as placing mental defectives in hostels while they received agricultural training, has resulted in several thousand mental defectives' successfully re-entering the community as self-supporting members.

Modern success in the rehabilitation of mental defectives is having a profound effect on life in those institutions where the work of reintegration is being actively pursued, and, in turn, on the attitude of the general population not only to the institutionalization of defectives but also to their readmission to the community. On the other hand, recent advances in preventive measures against mental deficiency have, up to the present time, been more remarkable for their morale-raising effect than for their actual contribution to prophylaxis. However, a considerable volume of inquiry has been undertaken, particularly in the United States, into the genetic factors and the environmental circumstances that may have pathological effect in connexion with pregnancy, parturition, and care in early infancy. Realization of the risk of maternal exposure in pregnancy to certain virus infections, notably rubella, and of the possible effects of metabolic disorders, e.g. phenylketonuria and ionizing radiation, has given a fresh impetus to aetiological research. The immediate advances to be gained from these measures as regards the prevention of mental deficiency are not at present appreciable, as may be judged by the fact, for example, that phenylketonuria is not anticipated more commonly than at a rate of about one in 100,000 live births, so that the provision of an effective prophylactic screen would be very difficult and expensive, to say the least. The real value of the prophylactic discoveries to date is in the enormous impetus they give to massive research effort. Tay-Sachs disease, a very rare developmental anomaly, is now thought to be due to an enzyme deficiency of glucose metabolism, and is potentially to be regarded as preventable. Other metabolic dietary and climatic factors are the subject of present inquiry (418). Pasamanick, for example, is conducting a series of inquiries into what he has termed a continuum of reproductive casualty, which extends from profound mental deficiency to minor subclinical conditions.

A more immediately practical advance, numerically speaking, has taken place in relation to the substitute care of children deprived of maternal care in early infancy. From the early work of Spitz, Goldfarb, Roudinesco, Bowlby, and others it has become apparent that a significant proportion of cases hitherto classed as defective or psychotic are showing a deprivation syndrome following loss of the mother when no adequate substitute arrangements have been made. Proper attention to preventive principles in residential nurseries and so on can hardly fail to make a significant contribution to the prevention of these conditions of infantile deprivation.

EPILEPSY

The principal developments since 1948 in the field of epilepsy have been in two directions: (i) improvement in the range and effectiveness of anti-convulsant drugs and reduction of disadvantageous side-effects of medication; (ii) greater integration of special treatment for epilepsy with general medical facilities. Modern drug therapy has made it possible for all but a small minority of epileptic patients to be stabilized and to continue to live and work in the community. It is now more apparent that what were supposed to be special characterological defects inherent in epilepsy were, in fact, largely artificially produced by the social and medical treatment of the condition.

In many countries it is reported that there are tendencies to close down special residential facilities for epileptics. In Australia, one special colony has been in existence for many years, but it is about to close. From Peru it is reported that special services were discontinued as long as thirty years ago. In the United Kingdom the use of special facilities for the treatment of epilepsy has been more than halved in the last twenty-five years, and the trend is continuing. In some countries there is considerable activity in terms of social measures for epileptics, including the formation of active voluntary organizations to provide sheltered employment and social supervision where these are still required. There remains in all countries a hard core problem of chronic epilepsy, commonly associated with mental disorder or mental deficiency.

DELINQUENCY

Although at the time of the Study Group (1961) there was probably no topic in the social field of more immediate concern in most countries than that of juvenile delinquency, there is very little to report, from the postwar years, of advances in techniques of care and treatment. The general survey of the psychiatric aspects of juvenile delinquency, undertaken for WHO by Bovet (316), has been brought up to date by Gibbens (318). The United Nations Organization has held a series of conferences on the prevention of juvenile delinquency. On the whole, the main weight of attention has been given to legal and administrative aspects, and while there have been individual pioneer efforts in education and community scientific research into origins, there is little to record. An interesting pioneer experiment in residential therapy for delinquent boys and their re-education in the community has been described (320).

Promising techniques for dealing with limited numbers of sociopathic youngsters have been developed in some parts of the United States, in the United Kingdom, Sweden, and a number of other countries. In Sweden, for instance, there has been a good deal of interest in attempts to raise the status of adolescents generally, and not only the delinquent minority, in the eyes of the community as a whole. It has been argued that the very term 'adolescent' betrays a somewhat belittling attitude on the part of the community towards this whole group, and has tended to provoke a relatively immature style of behaviour among its members. It is suggested that it is better to call adolescents young men and young women, and to offer them chances of participating in community life at a more truly adult level than youth movements have been accustomed to encourage. An example of this in Sweden has been the mobilization of youthful car enthusiasts into a club, which has a special badge and flag, one of the objectives being to give outings on Sundays to cripples. This project has met with some success in canalizing what might otherwise be quite harmful activities into a positive contribution to the community.

PSYCHOPATHIC PERSONALITIES

As stated above, there is an increasing tendency in many countries to deal with the problems of psychopathic personalities, which contribute to, but are not identical with, delinquency, by psychiatric methods rather than by traditional criminological techniques. We have referred in Chapter 5 to the potential danger to the image of the mental hospital in the community if doors are to be unlocked and the hospital more closely integrated in the wider community only to be once again used for the treatment, under duress, of psychopathic criminals. In a number of countries special state institutions have been set up for dangerous psychopaths. Some of these are run more or less on mental hospital lines, and in other countries hospital wings of prisons are used for such treatment or, alternatively, specially secure sections of mental hospitals. In general, recent developments in this field have not been of any great significance, but they have shown a greater degree of psychiatric orientation in the approach to treatment. Developments in electroencephalographic techniques have revealed the presence of dysrhythmias which may indicate that brain damage and structural anomalies contribute more specifically to psychopathic formation than has hitherto been thought likely. This evidence is suggestive only. On the whole, the community treatment of delinquency has still depended for its success on the therapeutic atmosphere of the community, and on the creation of positive interpersonal relationships within it, which can then be extrapolated into society at large. In the case of psychopaths this type of treatment has usually proved to be a matter of extreme difficulty.

MENTALLY ILL DELINQUENTS AND CRIMINALS
The related problem of those who are mentally disordered and also involved in delinquent or criminal behaviour has, in most countries that have made provisions in this field, been traditionally tackled either by psychiatric hospital divisions in prisons or by special psychiatric hospitals. Apart from a general recognition that psychiatric treatment could well play a far larger part in the rehabilitation of chronic criminality and recidivism, there are, in this field likewise, few achievements to record from the last fifteen years. It is widely felt by psychiatrists that duress is the least promising circumstance in which to start psychotherapeutic treatment, and that it is probably more effective to approach the task from the point of view of the therapeutic effect of community life. The lessons learnt during the course of the development of the therapeutic community within the modern psychiatric hospital appear to be highly relevant to this therapeutic field, perhaps the most difficult of all.

ALCOHOLISM AND DRUG ADDICTION
Alcoholism has been reported a serious problem in perhaps the majority of the countries that responded to our inquiry, and in many countries there is evidence of a considerable increase in

SOME MENTAL HEALTH PROBLEMS IN SOCIETY

special facilities, including outpatient services, for the treatment of this condition. Modern techniques of help are mostly concerned with treating what is now recognized to be the underlying personality condition that leads to addiction. Thus psychotherapeutic methods combined with measures of social care and control of drinking habits are the favoured approaches. Pharmacological methods, in particular the creation of physiological intolerance of alcohol by drugs (e.g. tetra-ethyl-thiuran disulphide – 'antabuse'), have had a limited application, but are recognized to be potentially dangerous in isolation because not only do they leave the underlying needs of the patient unsatisfied, but they can have a seriously depressive effect of their own.

Perhaps the most significant recent development in the treatment of alcoholism has been the emergence in a number of countries of self-help social organizations of alcoholics themselves often under the term 'Alcoholics Anonymous'. These are particularly active in South Africa and also exist in the United States, the United Kingdom, Canada, and a number of other countries. The types of social help that these organizations provide do not, of course, deal with the underlying needs of the patient unless additional measures are taken.

Drug addiction continues to present a major problem in certain countries and, as in the case of alcoholism, the most constructive development in this field has been the increasing recognition that it is essentially a problem of personality and that treatment must be related to the needs of the individual. The main weight of community action in the case of drug addiction continues to be in attempts to control the distribution of narcotics.

The Study Group recommended that the relative success of self-help methods as compared with more orthodox passive treatment methods in dealing with alcoholism and addiction deserves a great deal more study. It is clear that much in connexion with these problems relates to the comparative social isolation of the addict, an isolation that tends to be increased by punitive measures and attitudes which, the Study Group noted with some concern, appear to be somewhat on the increase in a few countries. Ultimately, the success of therapeutic measures must depend as much upon the morale and the self-respect of the people concerned as upon any other factors, an observation that may apply to delinquency and psychopathic behaviour in general, as well as to addiction.

8
Personnel Problems

In their survey of mental health conditions in thirty-three countries from 1948 to 1960, Krapf and Moser (5) have reported on staffing conditions, and a summary of their findings is given below:

1. Numbers of *physicians* per million population vary widely, from under 300 to over 1,100. Abyssinia and Afghanistan are at one extreme, with virtually no qualified physicians; Israel, with 2,260 per million population, is at the other. Increases of from 10 to 100 per cent are reported in the period studied, the greatest increases occurring in countries with lower numerical levels of staffing.

2. Numbers of *psychiatrists* per million population vary from less than one in three countries to sixty-nine in the United States. All countries show an increase in the decade studied, and several have doubled or trebled their number. It is noticeable that those countries with more physicians also have more psychiatrists. Figures are not strictly comparable between countries because of differences of definition and also different ways of presenting the data relating to mental hospital doctors and to other doctors.

3. Numbers of *child psychiatrists* per million population range from less than one in eleven countries to nine in the United States. Increases in numbers reported over the decade were up to sixfold. These figures are even less consistent than those relating to general psychiatrists owing to the widely different concepts of child psychiatry in various countries. In this connexion the recent recognition in the United States of child psychiatry as a sub-speciality for purposes of certification is the first of its kind, and greatly to be welcomed.

139

4. Numbers of *clinical psychologists* per million population again show a variation from under one in nine countries to fifty-nine in the United States, an increase being recorded in all the countries reporting.

5. Numbers of *psychiatric social workers* per million population vary from under one in six countries to seventy-five in Israel. Twenty-one countries provided data on this item, and most showed increases of up to threefold or fourfold over the decade. However, it is clear that the qualifications demanded of psychiatric social workers vary so widely from country to country that those who are recognized as such in some countries would not be so recognized in others.

6. Numbers of *trained psychiatric nurses* per million population range from under one in three countries to about 800 in two countries.

7. Numbers of *psychiatric attendants* and *practical nurses* per million population range from three in one country to 1,420 in one country.

8. Total numbers of *trained and untrained nurses and attendants* per million population range from under ten in five countries to 1,500 in one country. As would be expected, the countries with higher levels of psychiatric facilities have greater numbers of nursing staff. Increases over the decade in countries with low staffing levels have been small.

9. Numbers of *patients per psychiatric hospital doctor* range from over 200 in five countries to under fifty in three countries, but, again, practices vary widely.

10. Numbers of *patients per psychiatric hospital nurse* are over 500 in two countries, but under ten in five countries.

11. Numbers of *patients per psychiatric attendant or practical nurse* are more than fifty in two countries but less than ten in seven countries.

There were also large variations among the countries studied in the proportions of psychiatrists who worked mainly or exclusively in public institutions. The proportion was as high as 80 per cent in eleven of the countries that returned figures, and around 50 per cent in nine countries; in the remaining thirteen countries, psychiatrists generally devoted considerably more time to private than to public practice.

AVAILABILITY OF PERSONNEL

Krapf and Moser (5) commented that about three-quarters of the responding countries complained of shortages in all the categories of personnel mentioned. A major cause of difficulty in many countries is the uneven distribution of personnel. On the whole, physicians and psychiatrists choose to work in urban areas rather than rural. This, of course, is not solely or even mainly a matter of preference, since the difficulties of earning a living as a specialist in a sparsely populated area are very considerable. The United States return gives an average of one psychiatrist for 43,800 people in the ten most rural states, as compared with a national average of one per 14,500.

The reasons put forward by the responding countries for the shortage of psychiatrists include lack of interest in psychiatric specialization, lack or poor quality of psychiatric courses in medical schools, lack of psychiatric training facilities including training personnel, and the difficulty – linked with the above – of getting suitable candidates. Would-be trainees are also deterred in some cases by the prospect of low status, unattractive working conditions, and low salaries. It is widely complained that new services and specialist facilities are being developed too rapidly to be adequately staffed with the personnel available.

It is interesting to note that the return for the Soviet Union does not include any suggestion that psychiatric personnel shortages are acute in that country; psychiatry is included in the list of 'harmful' occupations and has certain privileges: e.g. psychiatric personnel have a shorter working day (six hours) and longer holidays (one month), and receive an addition to their salary of from 15 to 30 per cent, and various other benefits.

Krapf and Moser cite the report of the WHO Expert Committee on Mental Health in 1950 (23): 'in order to provide satisfactory treatment for all cases of psychological disorder . . . it is necessary for a community to have one psychiatrist per 20,000 population'. Only four of the responding countries approach this figure; in five, the existing ratio is something like a quarter to a half of the recommended level, and in others it falls far below. Even satisfactory overall numbers may not provide an adequate supply if distribution is bad; and the situation may be worse than it appears at first sight in many countries that have a comparatively low complement of psychiatrists should they, as is commonly the case, devote more time to private practice than to work in public institutions or services.

The Study Group noted that countries with low staffing levels have shown, generally speaking, a higher rate of increase in recent years in numbers of physicians; thus the most practical way of strengthening mental health facilities in such countries may be to expand the mental health and psychiatric content of the training of general practitioners – as has been done, for example, in Taiwan. In other countries, e.g. Peru, there have been attempts to compensate for the comparative shortage of psychiatrists by increasing the number of psychiatric social workers.

Shortages of trained psychiatric nursing personnel are described in some countries as 'dire'. These figures are particularly difficult to interpret because the proportion of institutional beds to population varies so widely. Where there are few beds, a high proportion of patients either are without care or are cared for at home; and it is a moot point which of these alternatives – care at home or care in a poorly staffed institution – is preferable for the patient and for the community.

Krapf and Moser (5) pointed to the 'catalytic' effect of even small increases in nursing force, especially if such nurses have been trained to pass on their knowledge. This has been the aim of many WHO fellowships and training programmes in psychiatric nursing.

NEW SERVICES

IN COUNTRIES WITH LIMITED RESOURCES

There has been very little systematic study of how to promote new mental health services in places where there is an inadequate supply of personnel. Hitherto, this situation has been tackled in various ways: by defining the most urgent problems and ignoring the remainder; by providing consultant services by means of which a few highly qualified people advise less qualified workers in limited skills in the field; and by various group techniques. Tooth (182), writing about a community with comparatively well-developed medical and social services, has suggested that psychiatric departments established in general hospitals should serve as headquarters for community mental health services, and should maintain close relationships with general practitioners, other medical services, and social agencies. Obviously, such centres would be on a small scale in many areas, but even a small unit can prove effective, provided that it is well integrated with other community facilities, whether medical, welfare, legal, or educational.

The Study Group considered at length the key question of the training of personnel for work in areas that are undeveloped from the mental health point of view (see Volume II, Chapter 11). Here, it will be useful to recapitulate some of this discussion where it concerns the practical organization of services. Taking the long view, the Study Group was convinced that in the introduction of new or more elaborate services it is essential to ensure that the future is not mortgaged by the creation of a first generation of workers with inferior education and skills, and limited outlook. Such action may cripple the proper development of services for a whole professional generation. In principle, it is advisable to allow local and well-established methods – however primitive and unscientific – to continue during the time that is required for the *adequate* preparation of new services, fully appropriate to the specific conditions and requirements of a particular country or community. The complete absence of hospitals or psychiatric personnel, for a somewhat longer period, is preferable to the more immediate provision of services which are locally and culturally inappropriate.

These views are essentially in agreement with those stated by the WHO Expert Committee in its tenth report, 'Programme Development in the Mental Health Field' (391), as follows:

'The setting up of programmes for mental health promotion, prevention of mental illness, treatment of the mentally disturbed, rehabilitation, and the education and training of personnel for the different services must be adapted to the special needs and to the available and potential resources of each nation or area. . . .

'Creation of new mental health services, or expansion of existing ones, should be postponed until a nucleus of trained professional personnel is available. To make temporary arrangements in the hope that they may be abandoned when more competent ones becomes available is not realistic. . . .

'Some of the local means of handling the problem, or of neglecting it in a socially acceptable way, have often been in operation for many years. To allow them to continue during adequate preparation for new services may seem harsh, but in the long-term view may be the best way finally to solve the problem.'

The point is well appreciated, for example, by psychiatrists working in Nigeria (73, 74, 228), on the Gold Coast (now Ghana) (85), and in the Sudan in particular, in connexion with practitioners of indigenous systems of healing and with 'treatment centres' (81). The Study Group was informed that in the Sudan there had been pressure to secure the banning of traditional healers, but this was resisted on the grounds that so great a void would have been created that there would have been far more intense pressure on the World Health Organization, or some other body, to provide a replacement which was manifestly impracticable – namely, a health service for everyone in the country. This view – that when circumstances are such that a long time is bound to elapse before modern health services can be provided for all of the people it is wiser to permit the traditional systems to continue – can be justified on the additional grounds that to banish the old system may endanger the introduction of a new mental health service through the arousal of public anxiety and, therefore, of opposition. But if the leaders of the community realize that the establishment of a mental health clinic does not mean that 'everything else has to go' then all may be well.

Prince (228) found that 'the Nigerian almost invariably preferred to consult the native doctor for psychiatric illness', and that almost all the patients attending a psychiatric clinic in Western Nigeria had, in fact, been previously treated by indigenous practitioners. This was true even of 'highly westernized patients who were aware that European psychiatric help was available'. African psychiatrists have thus been led, as stated by Lambo (74),

'to recognise the part played by indigenous psychotherapeutic approach in the total management of the patient, without any lowering of standard of medical practice. Even though by western standards this approach is inexcusable and some of the indigenous cultural factors may be caricatured as primitive and antediluvian, they are nevertheless emotionally reinforced and, as an historical and traditional legacy, the psychiatrist working in this cultural setting must be sensitive to their implications and reckon with them.'

Lambo (74) further states: 'In our village system at Aro, the native religious leaders play a conspicuous part in the psychotherapeutic management of some of the patients.'

Members of the Study Group suggested that, in the early stages of establishing mental health services in countries without psychiatric facilities, primary concern should be attached to the provision of shelter for psychotic patients, in the form of a simple, protective, non-oppressive environment appropriate to the particular culture, with kindly and informed nursing care. This phase would be followed by the gradual development of medical services, when suitably trained psychiatric personnel, financial and other support, and adequate organizational facilities might ultimately become available.

In 1950 Tooth published a report (85) on mental illness in the Gold Coast (this study was carried out in the decade before the Gold Coast emerged as the independent state of Ghana). He remarked that a visit to the local mental hospital, as it then was, 'should convince an impartial observer that the Africans' lack of confidence in the European management of this branch of medicine is well founded'. He recommended that until a sufficient number of African-trained psychiatrists were available it would be better to allow the care of the majority of the insane to remain in non-medical hands; and that the normal lines of authority in the community, emanating from the chieftain system, should be used for whatever restraint of psychotic behaviour might be found necessary. Tooth's further recommendation that 'observation compounds' should be built and staffed by local people who had had a period of training in the mental hospital was not, in fact, followed up. The intention was to create a somewhat segregated community 'to provide permanent quarters and occupation for the homeless, but harmless, chronic lunatics and to house borderline cases while their relatives were found'. This suggestion was modelled on the camps provided by the Trypanosomiasis Organization for the care of mental patients, 'trypanosomiasis being probably the commonest cause of mental derangement throughout large areas of Western Africa'. In this scheme there was a frank element of segregation and compulsion, and it involved the creation of a type of institution virtually unknown in the community and modelled, though remotely, on the plans of the isolation hospital familiar in Europe and America. It apparently did not find support among the people.

The African psychiatrist in the Study Group, commenting on the failure of this idea, emphasized that nevertheless there is an undoubted need for provision of some kind in many parts of Africa, where there is no one to care for sufferers from mental illness. One might go further and add that all over the world can be found individuals with varying degrees of social deviation, who might or might not be suffering from severe mental disorder, and who are in need of, and in some cases manage to find, some kind of refuge or sheltered position in the community. In 'Mental Health and Value Systems' (41) some discussion can be found of the attitudes in society to behaviour that is considered abnormal but not recognized as insane. Societies appear to have evolved a variety of ways of dealing with the eccentrics, the vulnerable, and the disturbed. They may be sheltered or persecuted or left alone; ignored; tolerated and allowed to live their own lives; assisted; rehabilitated; segregated; or recognized but neglected and allowed to die. The discussion (41) continues:

'Examples of social institutions that shelter eccentric, vulnerable, and disturbed members of the community have been found in many societies and at many periods of history. In the Christendom of the Middle Ages, religious communities played a very important function in this regard, both giving shelter to such people by design and also inadvertently by finding a way of life for many eccentric individuals. Religious communities in many parts of the world and of many religions are still serving this function.

'In many rural societies it is characteristic of village life that a small number of eccentrics are sheltered by the community and not only left undisturbed, but also may be found useful employment within their limitations. Among the industrialized countries of the West it is commonly found that large organizations also will find employment for a few individuals who are regarded by everyone as being not quite socially responsible, but who are tolerated as members of the community for various reasons. At another level, it is also found that universities, libraries, museums, and some other places with highly specialized functions can include incidentally a few eccentric people, who thus can contribute out of their strength, without being required to compete in society when their weaknesses might disqualify them.

'There have been innumerable examples of the more passive toleration of eccentric, vulnerable, and disturbed people in society. A common solution is more or less organized vagrancy – the "tramp" or "hobo". In sixteenth-century England the Poor Law provided food and shelter for vagrants in return for a prescribed amount of work. In Western countries generally it is usual for Authority to turn a blind eye to vagrancy, provided that laws are not openly flouted. In Islam religious mendicants are tolerated by society and allowed to live in freedom. In India, too, religious mendicancy may be a "shelter", and a particularly interesting example is that of the Senyussi, people who have taken to the jungle for a variety of reasons and live there an unorganized existence outside the pale of society but supported by the religious feeling of neighbouring communities.

'The attitude of society to psychotic behaviour and the treatment given to eccentric, vulnerable, and disturbed members are important considerations in any programme which includes among its aims that of getting psychiatric treatment started early, and which may raise the possibility of removal of the individual from the community. When psychiatric work is introduced into a community where little has been done previously, there may be some danger of invading the sheltered position of the people whom it is intended to help, without compensating them for what they have lost. When some interference in the life of an individual is contemplated in the supposed interests of mental health, it seems that at least the true interests of the individual demand some investigation of the degree to which his eccentricity contributes to his social conduct and his work performance. It is also important to estimate the amount of harm that his eccentricity will do to his work and to his relations with his colleagues and neighbours. It is possible to conceive of many positions in literary and cultural life as suggested above, which may be held by very eccentric people without harm, but with contributions which might not have been made by more "normal" people.'

There was some difference of opinion in the Study Group as to how far, in countries with very limited psychiatric facilities, this type of culturally integrated tolerance and protection of deviant individuals by a community, whether through assimilation or a kind of 'symbiotic' relationship, might, in the absence of specific local knowledge, be regarded as an adequate method of dealing with the more severe cases of mental disorder.

A psychiatrist who had recently undertaken, on behalf of WHO, a survey of the mental health services and mental illness in Thailand, reported that in that country shelters associated with Buddhist monasteries and psychiatric hospitals exist side by side, but it seems likely that, as the services become more and more oriented towards the Western European and North American pattern, the monastery shelters will tend to develop in a similar direction. He observed that, even in countries with highly developed psychiatric services, there are still many areas of need that have not been dealt with; and in the less-developed countries there are huge 'reservoirs' of human misery which have not even been recorded, much less appreciated. The survey of Thailand revealed the existence of many tens of thousands of schizophrenics who are not functioning in the ordinary social situation, of roughly twice that number of mental defectives, and of 100,000 drug addicts – all these in a comparatively small country with a population of some twenty-six million people.

This psychiatrist felt that some of the emphasis that has been placed on change as a cause of social tension might more realistically be laid on the reservoir of mental ill health that already exists in the community that is changing. He cited as an example the misery brought to a family where there is mental illness as a result of social pressures. Although individuals may *seem* to be functioning reasonably in a given community, it is possible that a great deal of mental illness is hidden, especially in the case of rural areas even in countries with highly developed services.

An anthropologist expressed concern lest this statement should appear to subscribe to the assumption, for instance, that drug addicts are miserable wherever they may be, and necessarily require treatment; or that psychiatry as it has developed in Western Europe and North America is what ought to be provided in other countries. These assumptions had not been intended, and it is well recognized that other forms of social and medical handling, other divisions of professional function, and alternative classifications of experience are possibly more relevant in other societies. Lambo, from his experience in Nigeria, concurs with this warning:

'In planning and organising mental health services, psychiatry in underdeveloped countries could profit considerably from avoiding the mistakes already committed in very advanced countries of the world. When we, however, try to abstract a lesson from European and American experience we must make sure that it will apply in the contemporary African situation. This is no easy matter, and we are getting more and more convinced that an independent diagnosis of our position may prove more profitable in the end than a borrowed remedy.'

On this point the Study Group was in emphatic agreement: thus the specific discussion reported above on conditions in Thailand must not be taken as an expression of opinion that it is desirable for a proportion of the Thai budget to be devoted to developing the best and most modern psychiatric services on the European and American pattern. In fact, the view of the Study Group is quite the contrary, because it appears obvious that it is not necessarily the same categories of people in different countries that are in need of treatment. Or, to take another example, in the case of India it would be ridiculous to feel a compulsion to seek out all the schizophrenics who are wandering around among the religious mendicants and put them in mental hospitals, without considering whether they might be happier and better adjusted as they are. On the other hand, it is equally unjustifiable to go to the other extreme and to behave as if these 'reservoirs of misery' do not exist.

In summary, therefore, the Study Group came to the general agreement that there is no evidence to justify looking upon the practices of those countries with the most developed mental health services and research facilities as if they constitute a kind of universal blueprint, widely applicable to other countries. There is little to suggest that people elsewhere would be substantially benefited by the provision of unmodified European-American types of service. In communities where the mental health services are undeveloped, the mentally ill might perhaps fare as well by being allowed to remain in the conditions in which they are happiest or best adjusted socially, at least until there is more specific and more locally valid knowledge of mental hospital treatment.

The people of countries where there is great need and where there are only very limited facilities for the treatment of the mentally ill should be forewarned against the adoption of any single and exclusive approach to the problems created by mental disorder, however strong the attraction may be in terms of high immediate gains through demonstrable results. For example, services based exclusively on one particular empirical form of treatment such as pharmacotherapy or some other physical method, or solely on a psychological approach, may prove to be exceedingly undesirable in the long run. They may, in addition, carry with them a danger of blocking more balanced development for an indefinite period of time, because the attainment of immediate results, however incomplete, may inhibit further effort.[1]

The above comment should not be taken to apply necessarily to the importation of some well-developed type of therapeutic practice supported by the full authority of a modern treatment centre, under strictly controlled conditions, provided that full account has been taken of cultural applicability (e.g. pharmacotherapy, accompanied by the establishment of a fully organized outpatient clinic with an interdisciplinary team).

Further, it was considered that it may be an effective interim device to add to those traditional healing practices that are already associated with the use of indigenous herbs and medicines some of the psychotropic drugs that have proved their value. This may help to pave the way for the later introduction of other aspects of a well-rounded mental health service.

[1] One example, among others, of the adoption of a single approach is provided by the new psychiatric centre established in Haiti, with the material and other support of certain pharmaceutical firms (82).

It is interesting to note, in this connexion, that it is only in the past few years that the effects of psychotropic drugs derived from several species of *Rauwolfia* and their alkaloids (reserpine, etc.) have been studied systematically by psychiatrists. The root of *R. serpentina* has been used for centuries in India in the treatment of certain types of insanity; and this ancient remedy, 'rediscovered' in 1931, is widely and increasingly employed today by Indian Ayurvedic and Unani practitioners, as well as by allopathic physicians (218). Preparations of *Rauwolfia* are also used extensively today in indigenous healing practices throughout Southern, Eastern, and Western Africa (228, 234), for the treatment of psychoses; and it is reasonable to assume that this plant was already employed for this purpose in African folk medicine a very long time ago.

9
Mental Health Action in the Community

Throughout the period under review, those concerned with the promotion of mental health have, almost everywhere, continued to be dissatisfied with the image of mental health that is projected upon the public. In a working paper, Rees expressed the opinion that this was not so true of psychiatry, as distinct from mental health: psychiatry seems to be becoming more respectable in the public eye, and mental illness and deviant behaviour are receiving more understanding than was the case a few years ago. Rees pointed out that those people who are more closely engaged in clinical work in a wide field of medical practice are generally more in touch with modern thinking about mental health, and this greater degree of sophistication has been reflected in discussion of these subjects in the World Health Organization. At UNESCO, where the approach derives rather from education and natural science, the discussion of mental health subjects has tended to be more concerned with social and moral issues.

It may be the case that the improvement in the public image of psychiatry has to some extent been achieved at the expense of the image of mental health. In the search to get away from words that carry bad connotations, such as 'lunatic', 'insanity', 'asylum', and so on, there has been a tendency in many countries to use terms like 'mental health' to cover, imprecisely, the whole field previously covered by the term 'mental disorder'. (This discussion necessarily refers explicitly and exclusively to English usage.)

Some of the current terminological confusion that exists in Great Britain, for example, can be illustrated by the fact that the laws relating to the hospitalization and other treatment of cases of psychosis and mental deficiency have been consolidated under the term 'Mental Health Act, 1959', and are administered by the

Mental Health Services Division of the Ministry of Health. In fact, legislative activity, whether in respect of health generally or mental health, is traditionally concerned mainly with the prevention, treatment, and aftercare of disease and disorder. It follows that the term mental health has tended to become synonymous with 'activity in respect of mental disorder'. There is great danger that the primary aspects of true mental health work may be lost sight of in the shadow cast by mental disorder, and that the image of mental health before the public may remain an unsatisfactory one.

The Study Group was informed that similar conditions can be found in countries other than English-speaking ones. It appears that the answer to this problem is rarely, if ever, to abandon old terms and coin new ones. This has been tried repeatedly in the past, and the result is merely that the stigma attaches to the new term.

The Study Group discussed the suggestion that an attempt be made to improve the image of mental health by reviewing the major new achievements in mental health work of the last few years, with the aim of defining more clearly the refined conceptual and methodological tools that have made these advances possible.

A notable new conceptual tool that has come to the fore is the idea of positive mental health (31), which we have discussed at length in Volume II (Chapter 7). The Study Group was convinced of the very great value of the idea that prompts the 'positive' approach but expressed some criticism, on purely semantic grounds, of the use of the adjective 'positive' (cf. p. 174 below).

A methodological tool new to this area is that of interdisciplinary action. Introduced into child guidance work rather more than fifty years ago, it is now commonly found in mental health research, professional training, and the mental health education of the public. Interdisciplinary collaboration is not, of course, the exclusive property of mental health action: it is common today in many fields of medical, social, and scientific work, but its very fruitfulness in the mental health field makes it desirable to consider in greater detail the complex question of cause and effect in programmes of prevention and amelioration.

Where there are several different individuals or agencies working together, how can the results of their action be ascribed to the particular contribution of any one of them, and to what extent? The answer to this question may be illustrated by the example of a witch in a primitive community, busy casting her spells and seeking to achieve certain personal ends. However, many other things are happening in the community at the same time, and when a particular event takes place – the death of a prominent individual or an outbreak of cattle disease – nobody knows for certain, including the witch, whether she was responsible.

The Study Group felt that the position of the World Federation for Mental Health was not dissimilar: that it is idle, if not impossible, to attempt to claim any result as specifically due to the action of a mental health agency. Perhaps the position of WFMH is more fortunate than that of the witch, in that the Federation may well rest content with the knowledge that it is reasonable to conclude that it has contributed to certain desired results, without requiring the reassurance of proof!

It is becoming clearer that it is more useful for the Federation to be able to create a favourable climate of opinion for its activities than to be able to claim credit for practical improvements or reforms that occur in the mental health field. We do not deny that there is an important scientific principle involved in the evaluation of action at the level at which it is undertaken, but the factors are so complex in this field that it has proved impossible so far to isolate the effects of any one agency sufficiently to satisfy scientific criteria. Until a more effective approach to the problem of evaluation is devised, it appears that WFMH will not be in a position to do more than make statements of what it has done in terms of simple reporting; that, for example, so many conferences were held, so many books or papers were published, certain information and other services were provided, etc.

It is far from simple to make even a straightforward factual report, because in many cases, although the credit for providing the initiative may go to one organization, a far wider circle of people is involved. For example, *Maternal Care and Mental Health* by John Bowlby (407) has been, since its appearance in 1951, one of the most influential publications in the mental health field; but, although its publication was entirely due to the initiative of WHO, the credit for what it has achieved must be shared among the people from whose work it was compiled, and thus must be widely distributed.

Some of the difficulties of evaluation have been illustrated by World Mental Health Year, in which a great number of agencies participated in addition to WFMH. When an attempt was made to assess results, it proved impossible to distinguish projects that had been initiated by World Mental Health Year, pieces of work that were already in existence but were brought into the ambit of World Mental Health Year by the people concerned, and activities that were purely coincidental.

It was pointed out at the Study Group that when people inquire into the cause of reactions or the results of activities they tend to think in terms of single causality – an approach, it may be felt, deriving more from a legal than a scientific attitude. Even in the realm of the physical sciences nowadays it is rarely possible to think in terms of single causality, and in the biological world it is virtually never possible. The Study Group thought that the principle of the enzyme might be used metaphorically to illuminate this discussion. An enzyme is necessary to many biological processes in that in the absence of the enzyme the specific process does not occur at or within the appropriate time. Strictly speaking, apart from its enabling or accelerating effect, the enzyme contributes nothing to the reaction and is not the cause of the process. It may be that the role of WFMH and other agencies in mental health processes is more analogous to that of an enzyme than to that of a contributing factor. The creation of a climate in which certain things can happen is, in an analogical sense, the role of the enzyme.

The Study Group agreed that an entirely new frame of reference is needed at a conceptual level for the evaluation of partial causality, a method that claims neither too much nor too little for such single factors as may happen to be identifiable.

It may appear to be easier to evaluate what has been done in recent years in the field of mental health services; but, though it is true that statements relating to actual advances in this area can legitimately be far more positive, the difficulties of assessing the influence of the measures on the community are no less. As discussed in Volume II (Chapter 7), there are both positive and negative aspects to be taken into account.

However difficult the task of evaluation may be, it deserves a more concerted attack than it has hitherto received from those who are leading in the field of mental health. It is a severe handicap to the realistic operation of a programme to have to do without the benefit of reliable feedback. Evaluation techniques are needed that are capable of taking account of the many ways in which voluntary agencies can exert a more or less indirect influence. They may be used, for instance, as consultative bodies – to suggest personnel for particular projects; or to nominate advisers on the mental health aspects of programmes. The influence of a single agency working through cooperating agencies may be spread widely through the sharing of literature; representation at conferences, committees, and commissions; nomination of speakers; and so on. The publication of reports and recommendations in suitable circumstances and at appropriate moments can have considerable effect on policy-making where it concerns the mental health field. This was shown with conspicuous success in the case of *Mental Health and World Citizenship* (12), which, it is believed, has had very considerable influence on the reshaping of policies in this field since the end of World War II. The Director of WFMH commented at the Study Group that it is known that nearly all of the seventy-four recommendations in that publication have been implemented in part or in whole somewhere in the world. There can be very few similar reports for which such a claim could be made, although the bare statement that the recommendations have been implemented does not indicate the measure of influence that the report has had.

There is current emphasis on the involvement of ordinary people in the community in prophylactic work and action. In Volume I (page 62) it is noted that in the state of Victoria, Australia, it has been estimated that half a million people out of a total population of three million are involved in some way, through various organizations, with helping the state mental health programme. In some countries, organized groups such as Rotary and other citizen groups have been helping mental health services in ways that they would not have contemplated a decade earlier. The growth of such ventures as marriage guidance and family counselling, which are now closely related to direct mental health work, is another indication of current trends in this area.

In many countries where there are active mental health agencies, a great number of requests are received from teachers, clergymen, nurses, child welfare workers, public health authorities, the courts, and youth leaders for help with the mental health aspects of the problems with which they are engaged. These are in addition to the existing channels of communication between mental health workers, general medical practitioners, and other medical organizations.

There is evidence that a vastly increased range of activities is being undertaken by mental health societies and cooperating bodies all over the world, a record of some of which was produced at the close of World Mental Health Year (8). The varied nature of the activities now widely considered mental health action is remarkable, and reflects a much greater degree of community involvement than has been the case previously. Another sign in many countries is that it is now far easier to get ordinary people to give their time voluntarily to work with patients in mental hospitals.

Perhaps the most significant of the new methodological tools that have come to hand has been the application of epidemiological method to the question of mental disorders. This has a bearing also on the more positive aspects of mental health because, in our view, it is not practical at the present time to define mental health satisfactorily in positive terms, yet more exact knowledge of the distribution of mental disorder would greatly facilitate the narrowing-down of the very broad concepts that are currently operative in this field. If the recent increase in legislative activity is to be kept on a sound basis, a considerably greater degree of precision of conceptualization will be necessary in a number of countries in regard to the treatment of mental illness. There has been a general tendency towards the repeal or at least the rationalization of outdated lunacy laws based upon segregation of the sick person and protection of the community's interests. Prevailing trends in recent legislation have been in the direction of making treatment more easily attainable and reducing the social disabilities of mental illness.

One major unsolved problem with regard to how to influence leaders of community thought and the people themselves lies in the degree to which it is justified to raise people's anxiety in order to get a response. Every psychotherapist working with individuals is well aware that it is valuable for the patient to have, early in treatment, what may be described as an optimal level of anxiety – enough to motivate him to seek treatment, but not so much that he is frightened off. The situation of the community is analogous though, of course, this problem is not exclusive to mental health work; in fact, it can sometimes be seen even more poignantly in cancer prophylaxis, to which the need to find the optimal stimulation of anxiety is highly relevant.

As we have discussed in Volume I (Chapter 6), it may be that some of the public criticism, and often hostility, to which mental health workers are accustomed can be attributed to the failure to strike a balance between frightening and motivating anxiety. The Study Group considered the notion that the irrational anxiety of members of the public contributes to the prevalence of the common smear that psychotherapy is 'brainwashing' – a smear that on occasion has included the implication that psychiatrists are concerned with teaching others how to undertake brain-washing for political ends. What is worse for the reputation of psychiatry is that psychiatric techniques and knowledge have been employed in a number of countries in so-called psychological warfare and counter-espionage. The fact that the overwhelming majority of professional people in this field have nothing but abhorrence for such prostitution of the skills that they have developed does nothing to neutralize the threat inherent in such accusations.

The least that mental health workers can do in self-defence, if they wish to continue to exert an influence on community opinion, is to confine themselves strictly to matters within their recognized competence. It is usually conceded that it would be appropriate for mental health workers to seek to help the leaders in the local community to make use of psychological principles in their work with people; and in some countries diplomats, politicians, labour leaders, managers, and other classes of leader may be of a sufficient level of scientific education and sociological sophistication to utilize these principles and thus come to deal with matters in a mentally healthy way. The resulting improvements will probably filter into society at many levels. But for the sake of their standing in the community, mental health workers must abstain from making claims of prosecuting a mass movement for the improvement of people, for the changing of personalities, and the like.

MENTAL HEALTH IMPLICATIONS
IN OTHER FIELDS OF HUMAN WELFARE
It may be useful at this point to enumerate those items in the literature that refer to some of the more interesting developments since 1948 over a wide field of human welfare activity related to mental health.

First, with regard to medical training, though the standard of psychiatric training in the general curriculum is, with few exceptions, very far from satisfactory, there is increasing recognition of the importance to the family doctor or general practitioner of an understanding of mental health principles: 253, 254, 255, 256, 257, 393.

Many publications have been concerned with the psychological welfare of patients in general hospitals, considering, for example: the reception and welfare of inpatients (262, 267); noise (262, 265); apprehension or fear (260). The British ministry of health published an interesting report on the pattern of the inpatient's day (264). The report of a study undertaken jointly by the International Hospital Federation, the International Council of Nurses, and WFMH was published under the title *People in Hospital* (259). It is the outcome of research done by eighteen voluntary interdisciplinary groups of general hospital personnel and mental health workers in Western Europe, Canada, and the United States.

Recent mental health publications in various other fields include:

Paediatrics: 280, 285, 291, 294.
Public health: 18, 153, 154, 207, 290, 327, 330, 343, 345, 393, 394, 395, 447.
Obstetrics: 249, 250, 251.
Psychosomatic medicine: 339, 340, 341.
Education: 16, 18, 439, 442, 450, 451, 452, 453, 454, 456, 457, 458, 459.
Deprived children: 16, 18, 424.
Crime and treatment of offenders: 16, 18, 316, 318, 424, 473, 475, 476, 480.
Human relations in industry: 460, 461, 462, 463, 464, 466, 470, 521, 533.
Accidents and prevention: 416, 428, 429, 430.

Of more limited but special interest has been concern about the application of mental health principles to work in the field of leprosy. Although the relevance of problems of mental illness to leprosy has been recognized traditionally – to the extent that it has been standard practice for leper colonies to make a high rate of provision for cases of mental disorder – in a letter to WFMH, dated March 1961, the International Leprosy Association drew attention to the almost total lack of workers with mental health training to be found in research in this field or in the rehabilitation of patients suffering from leprosy. The letter stated:

'Thus we feel that we shall get nowhere in the matter of leprosy psychoses until a psychiatrist can detach himself for a period from general work and study leprosy psychoses "from the inside". Such volunteers are urgently needed. . . . Most workers in general medicine are archaic in their attitude to leprosy, persisting in regarding it as a mystic curse . . . and refraining from taking the slightest interest in it as a human disease like tuberculosis or any other, even though it is probable that 15 million leprosy patients exist in the world today and perhaps one-fifth are receiving active care and treatment.'

It was suggested that existing leprosy workers might perhaps be sent to appropriate centres for training (cf. 334, 344, 346).

Another field of mental health influence that it is appropriate to mention here is that of community planning. There has been a great deal of interest in many countries in mental health and group psychological principles in relation to the planning of new towns and to community development. Thus there is now growing recognition that attention should be given to the emotional needs of people, as well as to the more traditional considerations in this field.

INTERNATIONAL APPLICATION
OF MENTAL HEALTH TECHNIQUES

Since 1948 there has been a great increase in movements towards national interdependence, whether in the field of intergovernmental action – e.g. United Nations, WHO, UNESCO, and other specialized agencies; or in that of technical assistance – e.g. the Marshall Plan, the Colombo Plan; or in the politico-economic sphere – NATO, the European Common Market, and so on. All these attempts at cooperation are providing valuable material for study from the point of view of mental health. Even more significant has been the experience of the emerging nations in the course of the process of gaining independence from a previous colonial régime. Where the colonial power and the new nation have been able to cooperate during the period of transition, the progress towards independence has, as might be expected, been much smoother than where there has been acute conflict. The questions are: what sorts of lesson can mental health workers learn from these experiences, and what can be applied to other situations in the future?

There have been striking changes in many countries in the attitudes of administrators to mental health matters – as is apparent, it was noted above, in the work of WHO. For the first half-dozen years of the Organization's existence, there were no national delegations to the World Health Assembly capable of making an effective contribution to mental health programme planning; more recently, there has been a marked improvement in this regard, and the spread of education in mental health matters, both within the Organization and in its external relations, has been rapid.

It is usually the case that success in international cooperation in this field depends to a large extent on the effectiveness of cooperation between voluntary and intergovernmental world, national, and local organizations. One of the great difficulties has been to align the interests of countries that have much to contribute with the interests of those that are mainly on the receiving end. A successful demonstration of essential community of interest was seen a few years ago when WHO funds were employed to bring a consultant in mental deficiency planning from the United Kingdom to the United States. The demonstration that a country like the United States, which is always thought of as a giving and supplying country, could nevertheless benefit from the technical facilities offered by an international organization improved both the feeling in the United States and the attitudes of other nations towards WHO.

The Study Group agreed that some of the more significant advances in the international application of mental health techniques have been made in areas not so directly concerned with mental illness. There has been increasing recognition of mental health involvement in a wider field of interpersonal relationships, and many examples of such involvement could be given. To select only three from the work of the Federation in collaboration with others: (i) the study of problems of human relations and morale in international organizations; (ii) the study of nutrition and the changing of food habits; and (iii) the study of principles of selection of personnel for work overseas in national and international organizations. These illustrations, and many others, reflect the growing awareness of the need to pay attention to mental health factors in the international context.

In a working paper, Torre suggested two specific areas in cross-cultural activities in which the psychiatrist is able to make an immediate contribution: (i) the evaluation of personnel for selection and work assignment; (ii) the training of personnel in aspects of interpersonal relations. In relation to selection, Torre drew attention to a fact that has been well attested during and after World War II in military and civil service selection processes and to some extent, too, in industrial concerns, that the social scientist can be of most use if he is a full member of the selecting team and completely identified with the project; that he does not serve as well or function as efficiently if employed in an advisory capacity. The field in which the psychiatrist's most useful contributions are usually to be found is that of judgements concerning motivation, anxiety and frustration tolerance, ethnocentric attitudes, adaptability to different conditions, interpersonal relationship formation, and communication. He can also give valuable assistance in the assessment of personnel efficiency and in the reassignment of experienced personnel.

The experience of WHO, and especially of its field programmes in the regions, has demonstrated that its role goes far beyond the purely technological aspects of disease eradication, though these latter are recognized to be vital. The carrying-out of nutrition programmes, malaria eradication, and so on has shown that the success of any measures introduced for the improvement of health depends on the way in which the human relations aspects are taken care of. There is an impressive body of experience, now, of unsuccessful mental health work – programmes that have failed because of the promoters' ignorance or lack of consideration of the effects of the attitudes of the people concerned. The point can be expressed in another way – technical knowledge is now sufficient to enable all mental health and social welfare measures to be introduced in ways that positively promote better patterns of human relationship and greater understanding.

We have discussed above something of the work of those voluntary, non-governmental organizations in the international field, whose roles have developed on lines complementary to those of the UN specialized agencies. In different countries there are various ways in which a voluntary body can act where the government cannot, ranging from one extreme, where the possibilities of voluntary action are not understood, to the other extreme, where there is a tradition that, whereas governmental organizations can undertake immediately only those measures for which the people are prepared and for which there is electoral support, the voluntary body is free to tackle what needs to be done irrespective of public readiness and no matter what innovations might be involved. In these latter countries the acceptable roles of the voluntary body are those of explorer, catalyst, and initiator. Further, in a number of countries a tradition has grown up whereby voluntary organizations initiate activities which, when they have proved their value, can subsequently be taken over by a governmental organization.

These concepts of the possible roles of voluntary organizations are not everywhere understood, and in many parts of the world it is impossible for any body of citizens to organize voluntarily without the active support of the government. In some cases there is no tradition of the citizens' taking responsibility into their hands for planning for the future; everything is left to the government. In other cases voluntary action may be viewed by the government as a threat to its stability or as an implied criticism of government inaction, which is therefore to be resisted.

In the field of mental health the difficulties that ordinarily exist between voluntary and governmental agencies may to some extent be augmented by those difficulties already discussed, which pertain to the nature of mental health work, especially the anxiety raised by the issues involved.

The World Federation for Mental Health is the most widely representative of the international organizations in the field of mental health. In 1963 it consisted of a federation of 139 organizations in forty-eight countries and ten transnational organizations; rather more than half of the members were interprofessional mental health organizations concerned with the promotion of diverse programmes of mental health work in their own countries; and the remainder were either professional organizations limited in their aims to promoting the interests of a professional discipline, or societies with a specific programme of work in a narrow field, such as that of retarded children. Owing to the varied nature of its constituent organizations, the function of the World Federation for Mental Health has been conceived of primarily as a secretariat and communication centre, and it has been thought possible for it to take on only small and highly specialized projects of its own. Since 1961 it has been found increasingly difficult to raise money for transnational projects.

It may be of interest to the reader to give a few examples of types of activity successfully undertaken by the World Federation for Mental Health since 1948. These activities may be divided into two broad classes: first, promotion of the interests of mental health work and mental health workers in the international sphere; and, second, support of work in the countries of member organizations. The former type of activity has consisted mainly of the organization of various kinds of meetings, conferences, seminars, and study groups; the promotion of exchanges internationally; and cooperation over a broad field with the various UN specialized agencies. The consultative status given by the UN agencies to suitable voluntary organizations has provided the Federation with opportunities to be represented at UN agency meetings, and to meet delegations informally as well as in the conference room. In addition, there have been many examples of cooperation in the holding of meetings.

Among the many meetings and small conferences that have been jointly the work of WFMH, other voluntary agencies, and UN agencies, with special mention of WHO, we would select here the International Seminar on Mental Health and Infant Development at Chichester, England, 1952 (510); the First Asian Seminar on Mental Health and Family Life at Baguio, Philippines, 1958 (*Reality and Vision* (434)); a conference on student mental health at Princeton, New Jersey, 1956 (453); a conference on malnutrition and food habits at Cuernavaca, Mexico, 1960 (483); a series of conferences on health and human relations in Germany, 1950 and 1951 (490, 491); a series of conferences under the auspices of the Carnegie Endowment Fund on human relations in international secretariats, 1957 and 1958; and a chain of study groups in eight countries on psychological problems in general hospitals, 1961 (*People in Hospital* (259)).

In addition, numerous other meetings have been conducted by one or other of these cooperating bodies, with full understanding in planning and mutual representation. To this aspect we attach particular importance because the impact and influence of these meetings are not confined to the matters exchanged or to the published reports, but include effects on world-wide cooperative behaviour between individuals. WFMH has also made contributions to the technical discussions in the World Health Assembly, and to various of the standing committees, working parties, and so on, conducted by that body. Similar opportunities have been provided by the other UN specialized agencies. Furthermore, voluntary and intergovernmental cooperation has been seen in the selection of governmental delegations to UN agency meetings that included representatives of the mental health point of view; this has enabled more informed discussions to take place on technical subjects.

WFMH has had meetings jointly with UNESCO, with the United Nations Secretariat in New York, and with CCTA (the Commission for Technical Cooperation in Africa South of the Sahara). In addition to meetings there have been study projects, and we would particularly mention the collaboration between UNESCO and WFMH in the publication of books on special subjects, e.g. *Cultural Patterns and Technical Change* (504), edited by Margaret Mead; and *Flight and Resettlement* (542), compiled by H. B. M. Murphy and others.

The Federation's own specific role at the international level has been to attempt to make original contributions to thinking – to the new conceptualization that is necessary in an era of great expansion of mental health work and of change. It was this intention that prompted the publication of the International Preparatory Commission's report, *Mental Health and World Citizenship*, in 1948 (12), and the subsequent formation of the Inter-professional Advisory Committee, to develop the original side of the Federation's work. This committee proved too big and too expensive to call together regularly and it was replaced in 1956 by a small international, interdisciplinary Scientific Committee.

The task of the Scientific Committee was originally defined as the preparation of working hypotheses that might form the bases of work in the future. The Scientific Committee set to work to produce a series of cross-cultural studies in mental health, with the objectives of seeking clarification, in an intercultural and interprofessional sense, of current concepts in the field of mental health that appeared to be emerging and gaining in importance, and of indicating areas for further study.

Cross-cultural Study No. I on 'Identity' (40), an attempt to focus current interdisciplinary thinking on this subject, was published by WFMH in 1957; it was reprinted in 1961, together with Cross-cultural Study No. II on 'Mental Health and Value Systems' (41), an inquiry into the compatibility of contemporary mental health concepts with various religions and ideologies. Cross-cultural Study No. III on 'Men in Middle Life' is an interprofessional study of the mental health, behavioural characteristics, and relationships of men between the ages of approximately forty and sixty years.

In addition to these three cross-cultural studies, the Scientific Committee of WFMH was responsible for preparing for and conducting the International Study Group of 1961; for the summary report of its work, *Mental Health in International Perspective* (*Prospective Internationale de la Santé Mentale*) (21); and for the extended report in three volumes: I – *Mental Health in a Changing World*; II – *Mental Health and Contemporary Thought*; III – *Mental Health in the Service of the Community* (the current volume).

Unfortunately, and to the great regret of the members of the Scientific Committee, the series of cross-cultural studies has had to be discontinued after the completion of the third, owing to lack of support. The Committee's view is that the technique that it has evolved, which is that of an ongoing study group, is proving very fruitful and is capable of considerably wider application, particularly in the fields of new concept formation and higher professional education; and that the withdrawal of this initiative from the sphere of international mental health action represents a considerable loss.

The second class of activity undertaken by WFMH – support of work in the countries of its member organizations – has been more diffuse and cannot be described adequately in a few words. It has been a primary task of the international secretariat, at first in London and, since 1963, in Geneva, to build up a sense of community among its member organizations, by means of correspondence, personal visits, and consultant visits, and by arranging exchanges of representation at meetings held by member organizations in their own country. An essential feature of the programme has been the annual meeting of WFMH, held each year in a different country with the local member organizations as hosts. Lack of finance has restricted the amount of travel possible, but since 1948 annual meetings have been held in the following cities: Geneva, Paris (twice), Mexico City, Brussels, Vienna (twice), Toronto, Istanbul, Berlin, Copenhagen, Barcelona, Edinburgh, Florence, Amsterdam, and Berne. In addition, during the same period, three International Congresses on Mental Health have been held – in Mexico City, Toronto, and Paris, respectively.

At each annual meeting, as well as the conduct of the formal business of the Federation, there have been papers and discussion groups focused on a selected theme (see bibliography, items 11–22). A particularly valuable feature of this series of meetings has been the formation, each year, of discussion groups in which a large number of participants have been able to gain experience in the interdisciplinary and transcultural discussion of mental health topics.

World Mental Health, a quarterly journal for member organizations and individual associates, published over much of the period under review, has added to the information exchange in this field, and regional conferences for members have been held in various parts of the world. On occasion, the international secretariat has helped a member organization to take on a useful piece of social service; the work of the Austrian Society for Mental Health on the acute refugee problem in 1957 and 1958 is an example. The WFMH secretariat has also cooperated with United States member organizations in two inquiries which have resulted in reports: first, on the selection of personnel for international, cross-cultural service (M. P. Torre, 1962); second, on attitudes towards mental illness, mental patients, and their rehabilitation among hospital staffs and the community (A. R. Askenasy and M. Zavalloni, 1963).

In pursuit of its primary objectives of education and promotion, WFMH organized World Mental Health Year 1960, when its constituent bodies in the various countries undertook a wide programme of mental health work, details of which have been published (8). The World Mental Health Year programme was designed in six main fields:

1. World-wide study of childhood mental health
2. Cross-cultural surveys of mental disorders
3. Teaching of the principles of mental health
4. Mental health in developing industry
5. Psychological aspects of migration
6. Psychological problems of ageing

Details of programming were the responsibility of the cooperating agencies. Activities included meetings to stimulate public interest, training schemes and research, and fact-finding projects. Some of the latter represented the inauguration of long-term plans, to bear fruit in years to come; others were existing projects, designated World Mental Health Year projects by their sponsors. A wide and varied programme was undertaken, some idea of the success of which can be gained from the fact that, according to information received later, more than two hundred serious research and study projects were launched in more than twenty countries as a result of World Mental Health Year initiative. Much more significant have been the thinking and planning that the exchange of information during the year has stimulated in many more countries. World Mental Health Year has been an excellent example of the catalytic action of an international voluntary organization.

Though the patchiness of the results cannot be denied, and some have been criticized as amateurish or even trivial, the protagonists of World Mental Health Year stand firm on the principle that there are many situations in which social action becomes imperative long before knowledge is complete. The application of this principle is not restricted to mental health matters; indeed, it is the traditional principle on which medicine has developed throughout the centuries; and not only medicine, but movements towards social amelioration and reform generally. Thus, in the mental health field, WFMH has judged it proper not to delay action until information is complete, but to go ahead using the best knowledge available, recognizing that much remains to be discovered and that mistakes will be made as well as successes gained. This approach is justified when those concerned are fully alive to the possibility of making mistakes and to the ways in which lessons can be learned from them.

This principle of pragmatic justification sometimes brings mental health workers into conflict with individual members of the professions concerned. As discussed in Volume II (Chapter 9), there are many areas of potential differences of opinion and attitude between those who are engaged extensively in the practice of clinical psychiatry, or in the central stream of the other cooperating professions, and those who are attempting to apply mental health principles to public work. Such differences are probably necessarily present, at least potentially, whenever work demands the cooperation of members of two or more professional disciplines. It is axiomatic that, whenever there is joint action between the members of two different professions, the field of action will be where these professions overlap and, therefore, mainly in areas that are comparatively remote from the central concern and core of expert knowledge of either of those professions. Thus interprofessional cooperation is inevitably a target of criticism of those who are narrowly concerned with their discipline as an exact science.

The major fields of cooperative effort so far have been: problems of cross-cultural communication, discrimination, and prejudice; the special needs of countries where psychiatric services are less highly developed; refugees; and the needs of moving populations.

10
Prophylaxis

In a working paper, J. R. Rees remarked that Adolf Meyer was heard to refer to some of his colleagues as 'mere treaters' – an expression that indicates the existence of a deep division of professional attitudes and suggests that, in some ways at least, the history of prophylaxis in public health is being repeated in the case of mental health. There has been the same progression of concepts, from those of segregation to those of active treatment, of social action, and, more recently, to some notion of building up greater strength. There has been the same sharp division in professional circles about the priorities to be accorded to therapy and prophylaxis respectively. Rees recorded a question put to him at the conference of the *Polski Towarzystwo Higieny Psychicznej* (Polish Mental Hygiene Association) in Warsaw in 1960: 'Is it true in any country other than this that psychiatrists are the greatest opponents of mental health?' The members of the Study Group were agreed that opposition to prophylaxis in mental health could be found to a serious extent among the psychiatrists of all countries with which they were familiar.

In recent years it has become customary to distinguish three levels of action in the prevention of mental disorders (392, 394):[1]

Primary prevention: prevention of what is known to be preventable.

[1] Various authors have offered alternative definitions, e.g.:
Primary prevention: all activities that tend to prevent the occurrence of mental disorders and difficulties.
Secondary prevention: all activities that tend to prevent the aggravation of mental disorders (e.g. measures to reduce the possible harmful effects of therapeutic practices).
Tertiary prevention: all activities that tend to reduce the return of mental disorders (e.g. aftercare and rehabilitation work).

Secondary prevention: the effective treatment of all identified cases.

Tertiary prevention: the identification and removal of harmful environmental factors.

To these three levels of prevention has recently been added the concept of so-called positive mental health (31). The Study Group strongly advocated the recognition and application of this concept, while objecting, mainly for semantic reasons, to the use of the term positive. The adjective positive implies a bipolar scale of variation – 'positive', through 'neutral', to 'negative'; the related notions of neutral and negative mental health defy definition, so that the term positive is unsatisfactory in application. Of the value of the positive concept, the Study Group had no doubt: it fully accepted the notion of positive factors in personality formation that could lead to favourable personality development, and of positive environmental experiences that could contribute to a state of affairs conducive to mentally healthy development. In preference to the term positive, the Study Group put forward the idea of 'optimum' mental health, defined as 'the best state of mental health that is possible in the particular circumstances'.

In considering the field of mental health, it is rarely feasible to distinguish between these four types of prevention as sharply as the classification implies. There are at present large areas of comparative ignorance about the identification of cases and there is a relative lack of precise knowledge about what is preventable; there are wide gaps also in our capacity to recognize harmful environmental factors and to identify precisely their related syndromes and the individual sufferer. It should therefore be borne in mind that a great deal of overlap is at present unavoidable in the discussion of these four types of prevention.

PRIMARY PREVENTION

Ahrenfeldt commented in a working paper that in the last decade or so very little of significance has been added to our meagre store of knowledge about the prevention of mental disorders. This is particularly true of so-called primary prevention. There is precise knowledge of how to prevent only a very few mental disorders, e.g. the pellagra psychoses and the mental complications of syphilis. Recently, some more or less precise information has come to light about the prevention of some rare forms of mental deficiency: e.g. it is now known that a fault in phenyl-pyruvic acid metabolism, which can cause mental deficiency, can be both detected and corrected within a few days of birth. But since the incidence of this condition may be something of the order of one per 100,000 live births, the immediate value of the discovery, though very considerable, is moral – through the boost it has given to research effort – rather than practical – in terms of the amount of suffering it may be expected to alleviate. It is known, again, that exposure of non-immune pregnant women to rubella infection during the first three months of pregnancy, whether signs of the illness appear or not, can be followed by the birth of a defective baby; but not only is the incidence of this form of deficiency very low, it is also obvious that the observations that have been made about this condition cannot be properly controlled. There is similar but less precise evidence concerning the exposure of pregnant women to extreme conditions of heat and humidity, or of ionizing radiation and so on (665).

There is more precise knowledge of the uses and limitations of thyroid medication in cases of infantile cretinism, but the mental improvement remains generally disappointing. Modern treatment of iodine deficiency is producing better results in the rare conditions concerned. Recent advances in haematology have enabled cases of Rh factor incompatibility to be dealt with by more satisfactory methods of serum replacement, which have reduced the danger of brain damage and corresponding mental deficiency. Refined diagnostic methods have enabled cases of galactosaemia to be recognized early in infancy and suitably treated by diet. The surgical drainage of internal hydrocephalus arising from structural defect and from meningitis is showing promising results. The successful antibiotic treatment of meningitis, and particularly of tuberculous meningitis, is another example of successful primary prevention of mental deficiency.

There has been a great increase in interest in the prevention of malnutrition, and of the deficiency diseases of women during pregnancy and of infants, particularly in tropical and subtropical countries. The main line of attack has been through education in child-feeding methods, especially at child-care centres (272). Geber and Dean (271) studied the psychological changes that occur with *kwashiorkor* and, conversely, the psychological factors in the aetiology of this condition.

Work on the effects of the separation of children from their mothers during infancy is now, in the opinion of the Study Group, sufficiently advanced to be treated under the heading of primary rather than tertiary prevention. Although admittedly the evidence has not yet been proved with complete scientific authority, yet its weight is such that no responsible person can afford to ignore it.

Bowlby's 1951 study (407) of the effects of maternal deprivation has been followed by several other interesting publications (409, 411, 414, 415). Main (173) has remarked that much less attention has been paid to the disruption of the mother–child relationship when it is the mother who has to go into hospital, and with this in mind has admitted small children to the Cassel Hospital, near London, together with their mothers when the latter have had inpatient treatment (cf. p. 80 above).

The concern that has been aroused over the question of the separation of babies from their mothers has raised the related practical issue of their substitute care during the period of separation. Following a report of a joint UN/WHO meeting of experts in 1953 (427), the British government published a report on the adoption of children (426) and introduced revised legislation in 1958.

The International Social Service (American branch) noted in 1953, in a report entitled *Experience in Inter-Country Adoptions* (422), that in spite of a marked increase in the number of such adoptions there was as yet no common pool of information at an international level about the results of adoption, notwithstanding the recognition that adoption required scientific understanding and professional skill.

At the request of WHO, Jean Macfarlane (440) investigated the use of appraisals of intelligence of infants and young children as predictive criteria in determining adoption policies. She concluded that such appraisals were not reliable during infancy, and recommended that prospective parents who felt that they could respond only to a child of high ability should be urged not to adopt an infant, but rather to take a child who has reached an age where prediction can be more accurate (cf. also 356). Recent experience has suggested, moreover, that the placement of a baby of inferior intelligence in a home of higher intellectual and social status than that of the baby's origin may result in an increase in the intellectual status of the adoptive child.

Finally, there is certain evidence accumulating about the prevention of schizophrenia, but not enough to constitute a proper basis for prophylactic measures. It is, nevertheless, being recognized that existing evidence justifies taking action now to prevent both the isolation of the aged and the institutionalization of the withdrawn or schizoid personality, and that such action should be regarded as being in the field of primary prevention.

SECONDARY PREVENTION

Among the few growing-points in the treatment of identified cases of disorder has been work in connexion with the theoretical and clinical aspects of family dynamics (431), including the diagnosis and treatment of disturbed family relationships; the effects on child development of mental conflict and family breakdown, and of 'neurotic interaction in marriage' (433). Pollak et al. (286) have written on the applications of social science and psychotherapy to child guidance work; and Masserman et al. (34, 35, 213) have published studies on familial and social dynamics.

The comparatively slow growth of child guidance clinics in most countries has been a source of disappointment to those who had hoped that child guidance would make a significant contribution to prevention. Well-meaning but extravagant claims have been made in many places that clinics would prevent mental illness and juvenile delinquency, but so far evidence has not been forthcoming of a marked reduction of the incidence of harmful conditions among children. It is plainly unreliable to draw any conclusions at this stage, both because we have little exact knowledge of the true incidence of the conditions concerned and because practically no successful objective studies have been made. The present state is far from satisfactory because, as Buckle and Lebovici (283) have remarked, 'although the importance of child guidance clinics is recognized by all those whose work brings them into contact with children, it is often difficult to ensure a place for them in national public health programmes'. In order to accelerate the development of child guidance clinics, then, it would seem essential to find ways of showing that those that already exist serve a useful purpose.

To plan and carry through an adequate follow-up study is undoubtedly a most expensive, time-consuming, and technically difficult operation. Owing to difficulties of establishing widely acceptable criteria of illness, presenting symptoms and signs, family aetiological factors, and the like, it has not been found possible to use clinic reports retrospectively. The same difficulties of criteria apply both to the course of the conditions and to the effects of treatment. It is necessary, therefore, to establish ongoing studies of children where the course of the disorder may be followed up by the same team, using a standard system of report-keeping and fulfilling the necessary control requirements. Whatever happens, teams will have to wait for perhaps half a lifetime – for the children to grow up – before the results of their studies can be complete.

Not least of the problems to be overcome in child guidance follow-up studies is that of appraisal of the true significance of the sample under study for the population as a whole. On theoretical grounds it may be stated, in the case of a service that is as incomplete as child guidance is, in every part of the world, that follow-up studies of clinic cases may reveal essential facts about the children themselves, but perhaps a great deal less of importance about the community.

Where new services are developing rapidly and where the personnel are insufficient in number and inadequately trained, the completion of proper follow-up studies has presented problems hitherto insoluble, a situation that tends to create a vicious circle of lack of public support for a service, the value of which cannot be proved.

A major aspect of secondary prevention now being developed is that of better and earlier case-finding through the education system. In order that this may be done successfully it is necessary to secure a greater degree of sophistication among teachers and parents about the possible significance of children's behaviour in school. Greater realization is needed of the fact that children develop at widely differing rates in the intellectual, emotional, and social spheres, so that it is imperative for the mental health of children to modify rigid age-staging for key examinations and school transfers, and to review the wisdom of rigid policies of school-entry and -leaving ages.

Modern prophylactic measures, especially in regard to children, are becoming to a larger extent a coordinated approach to protect both physical and mental health. For example, it is recognized that the discovery of a minor heart disorder in a child may lead to serious and long-standing invalidism if the heart condition is attended to regardless of the interests of the child's emotional development and attitudes. On the other hand, some children's ailments, such as skin troubles, which have been dismissed with a shrug, may need to be treated more seriously because of their potential effect on emotional development. Care has to be taken lest the measures proposed on 'mental health' grounds should conflict with feeling in the local society about the proper way to handle children. For example, although it has been amply shown that the most reliable way to improve the standard of nutrition of schoolchildren is to provide a mid-day meal at school, to do this may have harmful repercussions in the community and in family relationships, where basic community values are challenged.

One of the most striking recent advances in secondary prevention has been that occurring in the field of alcoholism and drug addiction. Mental health aspects of alcoholism were the subject of European seminars organized by WHO in 1951 and 1954 (302, 304). WHO Expert Committees have also reported on alcoholism (298, 303) and drug addiction (305). Duhl (296) has advocated studying alcoholism more specifically from the viewpoint of human ecology.

It is now widely recognized that the essential feature of the addiction problem is the personality disorder of the addict. This view does not imply neglect of cultural and social factors, which may have a determining effect in many cases. In illustration of this point, an African psychiatrist remarked that in certain tribes in Central Africa alcohol is regarded as a good and is used ritually by the whole society. In this case and in others it has been suggested that psychological abnormality tends to be found more often among those members of the tribe who abstain from the group activity than among those who participate.

Finally, in connexion with secondary prevention, it is found that as treatment methods become more effective there is a tendency not only to preserve and prolong the lives of handicapped people in the community, but also to save the lives of many handicapped babies who, under conditions obtaining hitherto, would have died. This situation places a tremendous potential strain on the families of the children and adults concerned, and it also tends to increase significantly the incidence of morbidity, both mental and physical, in the community. This paradoxical effect, combined with a great improvement in tertiary prevention, can lead to an increase rather than a decrease in the incidence of the morbid conditions that it is aimed to prevent.

TERTIARY PREVENTION

The great bulk of recent preventive action has been of the tertiary type, and it has been stimulated largely by the success of modern therapeutic methods. With the current trend towards the rapid turnover of mental hospital patients, who are being discharged at relatively earlier stages in their recovery, and with the correspondingly increased readmission rates in those countries where this trend is marked, the question of dealing with sources of environmental stress has become urgent. A profound difference has been made to therapeutic attitudes following the realization of the harmful effects on the chronic mentally ill patient of incarceration in a merely custodial hospital. It is now confidently anticipated that well-planned therapy, aimed at rehabilitation and social reintegration from the outset of treatment, will make a most effective contribution to tertiary prevention.

Current emphasis is on multidisciplinary cooperation, and on the need to spread knowledge of mental health principles among those dealing with large numbers of people – teachers, clergy and ministers, lawyers and legal officials; those strongly influencing community attitudes – policy-makers, journalists, business management, labour leaders; as well as among parents and the general public. This is not enough to constitute a full preventive programme. Soddy (278) wrote:

'Many types of preventive activity are undertaken: marriage preparation; antenatal, maternity and child welfare services; child guidance; special educational measures; youth clubs and movements; social welfare activities of all kinds. Even geriatric services are advocated, to remove foci of tension in families. These necessary activities help in the prevention of mental illness and maladjustment, but they do not represent a truly positive approach to mental hygiene. The difficulty about making practical mental hygiene proposals is that recommendations must apply to quite specific situations. Perhaps the basic necessity is that child-rearing practices should be appropriate to the culture.'

In many countries there is a strong emphasis on prophylactic work aimed at preserving or strengthening the family as a way of protecting both children and other family members against environmental stresses. The level of sophistication or objectivity of such work varies widely from country to country. At one extreme there may be a nostalgic recall of childhood memories of security in a rigid form of family life, characteristic of a traditional way of life that has long since been swept away by almost universal processes of social change. At the other extreme it may be fully realized that, where social change is radical and rapid, the true stability of the family is to be found in its capacity for constructive adaptation to change, and for creating new and living forms of relationship between its members. It is clear that, where there is a great deal of social change and population movement through urbanization or resettlement, it may be very difficult or impossible to maintain family cohesiveness, however habitual, whether the change is radical, entailing the movement of young parents away from their families of orientation, or of lesser degree, instituting a pattern of women going out to work daily or of men being away for long periods. Any such innovations will tend to raise stresses that would not arise in a more settled society.

It is now almost universally recognized that, if children are to grow up mentally healthy, not only must the maternal function be preserved whatever may happen to the family group, but it must be maintained in a way that is appropriate to the particular needs of the individual child in regard to age, culture, and his own expectations based on past experience. In times of change or other family stress, education of the mother for family living can be a mental health support for her that will have a beneficial effect on the whole family. In preventive work it should always be borne in mind that when the mother is not available, or is incapable of performing her mental health functions, urgent consideration should be given to the question of who is to give the family what it needs.

In therapeutic work there is an increasing emphasis on treating the family as a whole, without necessarily singling out for special attention that member who happens to be showing the worst symptoms. It is part of the more modern outlook to apply this principle not only with regard to the treatment of psychiatric problems of childhood, but also with regard to the occurrence of schizophrenia in a member of the family, and similarly of delinquency and criminality. In all these complex social preventive measures the cooperation of all people working in the field of social welfare is urged, and in no field more than that of marriage guidance.

The mental health problems related to the appearance of children in courts of law have been studied extensively in many countries. There is a widespread tendency to raise the age at which children are held to be subject to criminal proceedings, although in no country that we know of is there any measure of firm agreement about the age at which children should be held responsible in law for the consequences of their behaviour. There appears to be a general consensus that young children should be exempted from any formal legal responsibility. Many countries distinguish a phase of middle childhood, approximately from the eighth to the eighteenth year, during which children and their parents are required to bear a limited responsibility; and some form of compulsory supervision of delinquent and criminal young people is commonly enforced. In the Scandinavian countries, it has become the general practice, during the last fifty to sixty years, to remove entirely from the sphere of operation of the criminal law the public proceedings that arise out of delinquency and criminality among children and adolescents. The most favoured alternative approach has been to entrust the handling of problems associated with children's delinquent behaviour to citizens' committees that endeavour to do their work with the voluntary cooperation of parents. In certain classes of grave offence or in the case of persistent parental non-cooperation, legal sanctions can be invoked.

An interesting reform of court procedure has lately been introduced in Israel, whereby children involved in cases of sexual assault are protected by psychologically based measures when giving their evidence, and are not required to appear in open court. The Scandinavian countries have for many years protected children in similar fashion.

In the search for improved measures of tertiary prevention it would appear that nowhere has full advantage been taken of opportunities provided by the fortuitous occurrence of either natural or man-made disasters for furthering our understanding of the needs of children and adults under conditions of emergency. Thus it is a matter of regret that in the case of the severe flooding of the Dutch coastline in 1952, although the predicament of the children was handled by the authorities with a greater degree of psychological insight than in any comparable disaster in the past, little new was learnt about human reactions and needs in disaster, because sufficient skilled personnel were not available to study the situation systematically. Similarly, in the case of the Hungarian refugees and of other forced population movements since 1948, observations that could have contributed to our understanding of how to protect children in such situations have not been made owing to a lack of planning in this regard and a shortage of personnel. The valuable suggestion has been put forward, and deserves immediate implementation, that stand-by emergency teams of social scientists and of members of other relevant disciplines should be mustered, to be available at a moment's notice to carry out investigations according to pre-arranged basic plans.

The very considerable volume of work on mental health in industry that has been undertaken during the last half-century has been directed mainly at conditions of work and at welfare provisions, interpreted widely. But in the period under review the emphasis has been shifting towards the field of interpersonal relations, and has included study of the network of relationships between administrative, technical, and scientific personnel, floor management, working personnel, and the various welfare, health, and ancillary services involved. In particular, the industrial unit has been seen as an organic body, and, as the work of Jaques and his colleagues has shown (664), it is desirable that those who are studying an industrial situation should do so from within the situation and not, as hitherto, in the role of visiting experts.

As we have discussed in Volume II (Chapter 3), it now appears that processes of industrial change need not themselves necessarily constitute a harmful stress. Whether difficulties arise in the population as a result of industrial innovation depends partly on the traditional attitude of the community towards change, and partly on the speed and nature of the changing conditions. There have been a number of instances in recent years of communities passing from a peasant type of subsistence economy to an industrial economy, within the space of one generation, without evincing excessive strain. There is a need to understand more fully how this can be brought about.

One condition of successful rapid change appears to be the avoidance of what might be termed bad habits of living during the period of change. Bad habits of living are brought about, for instance, by the uncontrolled mass migration of a rural population to the outskirts of a developing industrial town, to live in improvised shanty accommodation, without water, sewage, or medical and social services. This has happened to some extent in almost every case of sudden industrial development in a previously non-industrial population, all over the world. Whenever a peasant community gives up its familiar type of existence for the chaos and hardship of the newly created industrial slum, bad results appear to be inevitable. It is now realized that social disorganization and disruption are not an essential part of the industrialization process, as has sometimes been thought in the past. On the contrary, with the planning and control of population movements, and with the provision of housing, sanitation, and public services at the same time as ensured continuity of employment, rapid and radical changes can be brought about in communities with minimal signs of strain.

QUATERNARY PREVENTION

Hargreaves (388) has remarked: 'In fact the best primary prevention may be the natural capacity of the organism to cope at a certain time or period of development with the presence of the stressor in tolerable doses.' This more basic concept of prevention, which has also been discussed by Gottlieb and Howell (375), is related to the concept of favourable personality development introduced by Jahoda (31) under the term 'positive mental health' to which reference has been made above.

The Study Group considered that it may be a very long time before measures taken to improve the natural capacity of the organism to cope with stress can be regarded strictly as primary – according to the definition given above – and, for the time being, the members preferred to regard this as the fourth type of preventive activity. This is a field in which there is, indeed, very little exact and established knowledge.

In a working paper, Soddy has written about the intimate role of the family in prophylaxis and has discussed what he refers to as the strengthening as opposed to the traumatic experiences of childhood. He points out that a great deal has been written about the so-called traumatic experiences that children may have, from those pertaining to sordid material surroundings to disturbances in family relationships and exposure to assault, violence, sexuality, and so on. It is well recognized that not every child is damaged by experiences that may severely harm some children, and it is proper to inquire what it is that makes a situation harmful to some, and under what conditions, and whether there may be other conditions under which a similar sort of situation could be beneficial.

It might be asked whether it is valid to take an analogy from pharmacology and to inquire whether there may be certain experiences which, like some pharmacological agents, act as a tonic in small doses and may stimulate growth, but are harmful or even fatal in large doses, or in different combinations, or in the case of certain individuals.

Soddy suggests that further knowledge in this field should be sought first of all in the intimate day-to-day experiences of a young child living in a family, and he advocates careful study of the relationship between family structure and behaviour, of the values and satisfaction patterns of the children, and of those interactions that keep the family structure constant from generation to generation. An illustration can be taken from a comparison of two widely differing styles of family life:

'The first example is that of the small, urban, apartment-dwelling family in an industrial area, in which from one to three children, somewhat spaced out in age, are brought up in the sole care of their mother, and not in daily contact with other adults or children, the father being present in the evenings and at weekends. The second is that of a rural family of four generations living together on the family compound, where the children are in constant contact with, perhaps, half a dozen women, and a dozen children within a restricted age bracket.

'In the first example, the baby's daily experiences with its mother are necessarily highly intimate and specific. Although daily life may be varied, its details are restricted and probably intense, an intensity which may include an element of hostility. For example, certain expressions on the mother's face, her tweaking of her baby's nose, her caresses and so on, are repetitive and acquire highly specific and often intense emotional significance for both parties. The child's adaptation to new experiences being at the hands of its mother, will be transferred to each new experience, including meeting other people. Thus the child who has an intensely satisfying relationship with its mother may be predilected to find new experiences and change both pleasurable and satisfying. But some element of rejection of and hostility to new experiences may develop, should the mother–child relationship contain negative attitudes, as well as the more positive.

'Another characteristic of families with a unique mother-child relationship is that the possibility of selecting between alternative courses of action may be presented to the child at an early age, and the child's attitude to making choices may get caught up in the maternal relationship satisfaction or frustration system. It is likely that although the child will value highly his intense personal relationship with that unique individual, his mother, and will reap the benefit of the reflection of maternal love in the formation of his own personality, he will also have problems of insecurity, inner hostility and aggression to deal with. This potential conflict situation may engender anxiety against which defences are necessary within the child's own personality.

'In the case of our second example, that of the child brought up in the family compound, circumstances may be different. Conditions will not normally favour the formation of a unique quality of relationship between the child and his natural mother. When half a dozen mother figures are present there may be little opportunity for the child's relationship system to develop on a basis of flexible trust and mutual understanding with any one of them. On their side, the mother figures have little opportunity to form, and maybe not the experience necessary to conceptualize, an idiosyncratic relationship with any one child. Since it is almost inevitable that an element of rigidity of common practice will appear when several people are handling children at the same time, the intimate experiences of the children may have too little inner meaning to the child to develop an affective intensity of their own. It may not become significant to the child who gives him food at any particular moment, nor who comforts him when he falls down. In short, multiple mother figures may bring to the child what might be termed the highest common factor of maternal nurture.

'Many interesting theoretical constructs could be submitted to examination: for example, is it possible that for the child with the unique mother relationship, personalities could come to mean more than actual experience; while for the multiple mothered child the form of life could matter more and personalities less?'

It is important to know more about what kinds of circumstances have what kinds of effect in various forms of family life; and what sorts of defences children need. Discussing the question of anxiety, Soddy suggests that

'the child brought up by a single mother figure, as compared with a child who has multiple mother figures, will tend to be more exposed to idiosyncratic situations with significant emotional tension. More may be expected of him as an individual, and his conduct may be more closely supervised. Because of the likelihood of less formality in daily life, there may be a tendency for greater exposure to choice-making situations, and although the rewards of success may be greater, the child will be more alone in bearing the consequences of failure. This combination of circumstances suggests that the child in the former example will tend to be exposed more frequently and more individually to anxiety-provoking situations than the latter.'

From this view it might be reasonable to advance the hypothesis that the more the child's relationship-formation depends on a unique mother figure, the more his defences are based on the quality and intensity of the interpersonal relationships within the very small family group. Thus the child's satisfaction in the parental relationship and in the new experiences derived from that relationship provides the main security in anxiety-raising and unfamiliar situations, a security that is based on the child's identification with his parents and, being carried by the child within himself, may be more or less independent of an environmental framework.

'On the other hand, the more a child's relationship system approximates to a multiple mother situation, the more the child's defences tend to be based on the wider framework of family life, the support of a range of family members and particularly that of activities and learning in common. Thus familiarity of the pattern of living is an important basis of security, and experiences that tend to separate the individual from his fellows may act as a threat. Adaptation to new circumstances tends, therefore, to be a matter for the whole community acting in concert, rather than for the individual.'

It should be emphasized that the contrasting styles of family life used in the above illustration are, in fact, a considerable oversimplification of a complex situation into a clearly dichotomous pattern, and the example is introduced only as a basis from which to ask further questions. Oversimplification though it may be, it well indicates the potential danger of applying the conclusions drawn from experience in one type of culture to another. An illustration of this point is offered by the social action that is spreading to many parts of the world in connexion with making provision for children who are deprived of their parents at an early age. The pioneer clarifying work of Bowlby (407) and others on the possible effects of separation of babies and young children from their mothers has created a great deal of public anxiety and has resulted in beneficial social action in some countries of Western Europe, in North America, and elsewhere, but has had much less repercussion in some other parts of the world. It may not be more than a slight exaggeration to remark that in some countries where these discoveries have been publicized the anxiety created has been such that many people appear to believe that it has actually been claimed that it is always traumatic to separate an infant from maternal care; the absurdity of which belief has undoubtedly increased the tendency of some people to reject the whole thesis. The objective fact is that Bowlby's studies have been made in a culture where the unique mother-infant tie is highly valued, and his essential contribution has been merely to find evidence that mother–baby separation is potentially traumatic when no adequate substitute relationship is formed, and may result in the child's permanent incapacity to live the type of life that the culture requires. There is nothing in any of this work to imply that the same conditions obtain in a culture where multiple mothering and an extended family relationship are the rule.

Soddy comments that in countries where the family structure has wide ramifications of relationship, the need for substitute care for children outside the family will obviously arise less frequently. In contrast, where the family group is restricted because there are fewer members of the family available to care for the children, the need for substitute care outside the family will arise more frequently; up to the present, however, it has nearly always been supplied in the form of a residential nursery, in which a group of perhaps twenty or thirty children of the same age are placed under the joint care of, say, half a dozen nurses. Thus, paradoxically, in a society in which the unique mother-child relationship is the standard, its breakdown tends to be replaced by society with a multiple mothering situation, which has little or no relevance to the types of interpersonal relationship that are characteristic of the culture.

'In a community in which the family is based on small autonomous biological units, such a residential nursery, standard pattern though it often may be, can have, it seems to be widely agreed, a very destructive effect on children's capacity to develop normally. At least in some countries an enormous effort has been expended in re-creating the small-family atmosphere wheverever children have to be cared for in the absence of parents. Inasmuch as the greatest strength of the small family unit appears to be in the intensity and detail of the intimate relations that children form with adults, such attempts can hardly succeed unless they provide not only the form of the small family, but also the atmosphere.

'It seems to be exceedingly difficult for an adult, or group of adults, to provide a satisfying but intense experience of emotional relationship on a long-term basis for other people's children. This should not be surprising, when it is reflected that to do so requires, as a basis, a loving partnership between a man and a woman, a partnership that is mutually devoted to the child. It seems likely that in many countries today, particularly in the West, a great deal of public money is being spent on what may prove to be largely futile activity, establishing small children's homes that give the form of a small family relationship, but not its true content.'

The Study Group concluded that, as these illustrations have shown, we cannot claim to be more than at the beginning of understanding the types of relationship and experience that will have a strengthening effect on young children in any particular style of family life or culture. Thus the true science of prophylaxis in this respect is itself only in its infancy, and constitutes a major aspect of preventive mental hygiene for study and action in the immediate future.

PART TWO

Research

II
Aspects of Mental Health Research

PRIORITIES
It would probably be readily agreed that the situation of research in the mental health field is nowhere satisfactory. In much of the world there is no mental health research of any serious kind in progress, and in those parts of the world in which a considerable volume of research is being carried on the position is at best unorganized and at worst chaotic. The Study Group thought that much human endeavour in this field had been applied ineffectually because of the general lack of agreed principles about what should be investigated and which techniques it would be appropriate to use.

We have remarked elsewhere that the prevailing scientific research methods in the world today have, with very few exceptions, been developed in the field of the natural sciences, and that the transference of such research methods to the field of biology in general and of human behaviour in particular is presenting certain serious difficulties.

Techniques of observation and study, using strict control methods, are difficult enough to carry out reliably in the field of natural science in working with inanimate matter, and they have only a limited application to the field of biology because of the living character of the research material.

When it comes to the application of controlled observation techniques to the study of human behaviour, the problems to be solved are extremely complex. We need only mention here the difficulties of identifying, isolating, and controlling variable factors, and the virtual impossibility of determining or controlling the conditions in which the group under observation is living. The technical difficulties of making strict comparisons between human individuals or groups are manifold. Although in loose terms the bodily and mental constitutions of two different individuals are identical and their biological rhythms very similar, their many variations of detail cannot be adequately allowed for; and their essential differences both at a genetic level and in their respective life experiences defy experimental control. These difficulties apply no less to studies of human beings in groups, and, though a greater degree of comparability can be reached by the use of immense numbers, the expense of such undertakings is commensurate with their size.

Not least of the difficulties of evolving genuinely scientific techniques for mental health observation and research is the tendency of scientists who have been brought up in the specific research methods of the natural sciences to undervalue and decry the efforts of those who are developing research methods suitable for the study of man.

The Study Group felt that, as a preliminary to working out precise research techniques, it is vital to seek a greater measure of agreement than exists at present on the urgency and priorities of research problems in this field. As a starting-point to discussions it was suggested that priorities in research be determined according to the following six categories (not necessarily in their true order of importance):

(i) the quantitative significance of the problem

(ii) the seriousness of its consequences to the individual

(iii) its social import

(iv) the existence of promising leads into research

(v) the scientific interest and technical resources that are available

(vi) the readiness with which public financial support can be found.

Of these six categories the last appears to be the least reliable, and the least related to the others.

How this system of criteria might work out can be illustrated by reference to recent metabolic research into the origin of certain diseases causing mental deficiency in children which has attracted great public interest and support.

(i) The quantitative significance of these diseases is very small indeed – e.g. phenylketonuria, the most familiar, is estimated variously as occurring in something of the order of one in 100,000 live births.

(ii) The seriousness of the consequences to the individual is, in most cases, profound.

(iii) Compared with other problems of childhood wellbeing, the social significance of these diseases and their cure is very slight indeed. Most doctors, even paediatricians, will not see more than two or three cases in a professional lifetime. Because of their rarity, even the complete extirpation of all the metabolic disorders at present recognized as connected with mental deficiency could not make any appreciable difference to the incidence of mental deficiency in the next generation.

(iv) There are a number of promising leads into further research with the possibility of major breakthroughs into new knowledge of the somatic factors in mental disorders.

(v) A considerable volume of scientific interest is now developing in these areas among biochemists and physiologists, but the technical resources that are available in most places are very patchy indeed. This kind of research requires advanced laboratory facilities and special training in areas that are remote from the psychological and sociological approach and even from ordinary clinical practice. The difficulties caused by shortage of trained scientific personnel are therefore augmented by those of communication between members of widely disparate scientific disciplines.

(vi) In comparison with the psychological and sociological approach, research projects in the metabolic area have commanded considerable public financial support during the last few years.

To sum up, projects of research into the metabolic origins of mental deficiency might be rated as follows:

(i)	very low	(iv)	high
(ii)	very high	(v)	low
(iii)	low	(vi)	high

The above attempt at rating represents an opinion with which, of course, not everyone would agree, but it is offered as an illustration of the way in which the rating system might be used by individuals for the clarification of thought, the encouragement of effort, and the restraining of unjustified enthusiasms. One cannot, for example, justify increased concentration on metabolic forms of research on the grounds of their immediate practical value to those affected by these problems, nor, strictly, on the speculation that valuable new curative techniques may come to light in the foreseeable future – though both of these claims have been advanced. On the other hand, the likelihood of improving the whole status of exact knowledge in this field will be held by many to be justification enough, and the encouragement that has been given both to research and to therapeutic personnel is an additional reason.

The Study Group agreed that it was hardly useful at this stage to attempt to spell out priorities in precise terms, but that all the above factors need to be taken into general consideration by research workers. It may well be a sounder basis for the award of priorities for the research worker to follow his own creative impulses. The history of research has shown repeatedly that some of the key discoveries have seemed at first sight to have no important bearing or practical implication – the classical illustration being the delayed but eventual discovery of the antibiotic properties of penicillin through the accidental contamination of a culture plate.

There are two interesting current tendencies in this field which deserve further consideration: first, research projects tend to involve more and more people of different disciplines and to need more technical equipment; second, the money available for research purposes is usually centralized and disbursed either by government or by voluntary agencies, such as Foundations. The tremendous advantage of this latter trend has been an increase in the money available for all kinds of scientific research; and the responsible agency personnel are, in general, very research-minded.

But there have been other consequences: for example, as research-granting agencies have proliferated and grown more influential they have tended to appoint technically qualified personnel, together, in some cases, with advisory groups, in order to evaluate the projects that are submitted to them for financial support; the object is that the agency should make its own independent judgement of the value of each specific research project.

This trend represents a very considerable change of practice from the days when it was more common for research money – admittedly in far smaller quantities – to be made over to universities or other relevant institutions, or to individuals of proved research capacity, in whose hands would lie the choice of the specific research field. This practice was, perhaps, less favourable to the new and unknown entrant to the research field, whose chances would depend upon getting the support of an established individual. However, it had the considerable advantage that the final choice of research project was made either by the scientist responsible or by someone close to him and answerable to the organization in which the work was to be carried out.

When a money-granting agency sets out to make its own judgement, it has to evaluate not only the ability of the applicant but also the soundness of the project and the usefulness of the technique. In the case of mental health, the field of research in question is relatively unexplored and in a state of rapid development. It is very much in need of a highly specific and *ad hoc* new approach and of relevant new techniques. It may be questioned whether either an individual who has left active research work or an advisory committee equipped to cover a wide field of scientific work is in the best position to evaluate new work in an unexplored but newly developing field.

We have encountered, in many areas, stereotyped attitudes

about what is respectable in mental health research models, attitudes that have been derived from other branches of science, even from non-biological science. When there is a tendency towards the centralization of funds for research, the effect of such stereotypes may be that research workers with truly original programmes fail to obtain financial support. In effect, the organizations granting the funds are determining the research programme as well, although they are not responsible for actually doing the work. Thus would-be researchers have to pick on a subject that will command support, that is thought respectable or is currently in fashion. The unhealthiness of this situation is that direction and control of their own work pass from the hands of the individuals who are at the growing edge of the subject into the hands of people who may have neither experience nor training, nor a personal professional stake in the work that they are now able to control and develop. Research programmes may be adopted not because they have engendered enthusiasm in the scientists themselves, but because they have won the approval of executors of fund-disbursing organizations.

The scientific policy of WFMH has, in fact, already suffered a setback through the effects of this modern trend. As noted above (page 168), the objective adopted by the Executive Board of WFMH was to publish a series of original cross-cultural studies on subjects of emerging importance. A later Executive Board added the rider that the continuation of the studies should be contingent upon project money being forthcoming from fund-granting agencies. Unfortunately, the agencies were not interested in the programme and the series had to be abandoned in the course of the third study on 'Men in Middle Life'. Thus, whoever it may be who is directing the Federation's scientific policy, it was not, in this instance, the Federation itself.

Another reason why the centralization of research funds has militated against the financing of original mental health research is because mental health research workers tend to be denigrated by those in other fields of scientific research – to a serious extent in various parts of the world. Not only is the behavioural science investigator regarded as 'unscientific' – an attitude that natural scientists extend towards a wide field of social science research – but there is a more general tendency for natural scientific opinion to value the research worker according to the material on which he is working.

Not only the research worker, but also the clinician may suffer from such negative attitudes of natural scientists. Thus the clinical research worker may be held to be unscientific because so much of his research field, being affected by human behaviour, cannot be controlled, in the strict scientific sense. In the case of mental health research, there is an additional factor: it is quite commonly held, and not entirely as a joke, that those who take up psychiatry as a profession are slightly eccentric themselves – or may be mad – and the desire to undertake research into psychiatry is held to indicate a morbid state of curiosity.

An anthropologist remarked on a tendency of scientific opinion to downgrade the research worker who deals with denigrated people. Thus the research worker in the field of mental retardation may himself be regarded as being less bright than his opposite number in medical clinical research; those who work on homosexuality may be suspected of being homosexuals themselves; and, more explicitly, those who work on sex may be regarded as pornophiliac; people who work on alcoholism are sometimes suspected of doing so as a defence against their own alcoholic tendencies; and so on. (It may be remarked that, since the clinical pathologist does not often appear to be regarded as coprophiliac, nor the morbid anatomist as necrophiliac, the stigma is a selective one!)

After considerable discussion, the Study Group decided that the situation is far too complex, and knowledge of the various conditions and possibilities far too sketchy, to justify any attempt to indicate research priorities in any part of the world. The most it is reasonable to do is to point to a few areas of particular interest in the world today that are outside the more strictly clinical types of research; the significance of the latter is of a different order and needs highly specific consideration.

There are, in the wider field, a number of burning social issues in which human relations are involved: e.g. the mental health aspects of intergroup relations; technical assistance programmes and the sudden and extensive technological changes that are taking place in many countries, with all their mental health implications; the spread of automation; the question of the peaceful uses of nuclear energy; and so on. In many countries the need is felt to know far more about the various forms of mental ill health and to define more precisely their relation to eccentric behaviour. To all these problems the application of modern social study and of epidemiological methods is, we believe, of first importance.

In a country where the development of psychiatric services is new, it is particularly desirable that a research element be included from the beginning of planning. In this connexion a psychiatrist suggested that a high priority be given to: (i) the recording of mental illness data, using the diagnostic terminology of the country concerned, with a view to compiling incidence and prevalence records; (ii) statistically controlled studies of the incidence of mental deficiency, with aetiological research in mind; (iii) the application of social research methods both to educational plans and to the interim results of new developments in education; and (iv) the application of social research methods to study what happens to the mentally ill in a community that gets involved in changing conditions, and what results may accrue.

DEVELOPMENT STUDIES

In some ways the last two or three decades might be regarded as the golden age of long-term studies of human development, and many references to these studies can be found in the literature. More recently, a great deal of interest in developmental research has been aroused by a number of conferences, notably the International Seminar on Mental Health and Infant Development at Chichester, England, in 1952 (510); the WHO study groups on the psychobiological development of the child, 1953-56 (279); and the First Asian Seminar on Mental Health and Family Life at

Baguio, Philippines, in 1958 (434). Reference should also be made to the CCTA/CSA report on the psychology of African and Madagascan populations (512); and to the study by Geber and Dean (497) on psychomotor development in African children.

The disadvantages that research workers tend to suffer if they undertake research into an area which is socially denigrated, a psychiatrist suggested, could be avoided in the case of retarded and aberrant forms of development if the focus of the research were placed on maturation and development patterns.

A psychologist from Africa wished to see more specific, longitudinal studies undertaken into the effects of environmental circumstances on human development: e.g. the effects of malnutrition on children, and the later effects of certain child-rearing practices. He drew attention to the existence of a number of critical stages in maturation patterns. There is some evidence that in the case of certain cognitive and motor skills there is a critical period in development when the individual is most responsive to training. Training provided subsequent to the optimum stage of maturation may be much less effective. This has often given rise to impressions that certain groups or communities possess an innate incapacity for acquiring particular skills. It is now thought more likely that their incapacity is mainly the accident of circumstances that have prevented them from acquiring the essential habits on which the subsequent more highly patterned skills are based.

This psychologist remarked that much of the work done on human development today is strongly under the influence of Gesell's studies of norms, although it is now realized that not only are these norms highly specific to the group from which they were derived, but, as Gesell himself has shown, they are in a state of continuous change within that group. It may be expected that, when a set of norms is the only one published in a field of work, it will acquire a reputation for general validity that far exceeds the fact; but the distortion that may be caused by its uncritical acceptance is a matter of considerable concern to research workers. Geber and Dean (497) have shown that, in comparison with the Gesell norms, a sample of African children was very much advanced in most aspects of development in the first year, but that the general curve of development of these children crossed the Gesell curve in the second year and thereafter the respective rates of development of the two samples were more or less unrelated. There are in progress a number of developmental studies in Africa – in Ghana, Nigeria, Uganda, and South Africa – and all are strongly influenced by the Gesell approach. Inasmuch as the Gesell norms are strictly related to and assessed in terms of the child-rearing practices of the group to which they refer, it is not objectively scientific to attempt to make comparisons of various groups of African children by such means.

In view of public concern, particularly in the countries of Western Europe and North America, with the behaviour problems of adolescence and juvenile delinquency, the importance of relating the psychosocial phenomena of adolescence to both earlier and later stages of development is self-evident. The field of work here is vast and complex – but as a limited practical suggestion the Study Group thought that it would be profitable to supplement very valuable current work with studies on the separation of fathers from their families and on the effects of such separation – for varying periods and in varying circumstances – on child development at different ages and in different patterns of family life.

AETIOLOGY AND PATHOLOGY OF MENTAL DISORDERS
This vast field of research is at present characterized by great activity but also by a general lack of coordination of organization. Recent research has thrown little additional light on the aetiology and pathology of mental disorders, and it is doubtful whether very much headway will be made in this field until there is a wider acceptance, as Krapf has pointed out, 'of the integral view of the disorders of the brain and of the personality which is . . . the most significant acquisition of recent research in psychiatry' (332).

Some Soviet psychiatrists have undertaken research on the aetiology of schizophrenia, on a hypothesis that it is a virus disease (377). Scandinavian investigators, on the other hand, have undertaken a series of genetico-statistical studies of schizophrenia, mental deficiency, hysteria, and involutional melancholia (106, 315, 333), in an attempt (with inconclusive results so far) to discover more about the role of genetic factors in these diseases.

We have been impressed by the potential significance for the understanding of mental disorders of recent work by Lidz, Fleck, and others (348, 349, 350) on the role of family dynamics in schizophrenia; and by Gibson et al. (314) on the pathogenesis of epileptic and hysterical seizures.

In the field of subnormality the genetic basis of mongolism has been established by the recent discovery of an extra chromosome in the cells of affected individuals, although the cause of this abnormality remains unknown (660).

For a useful source of information on various aspects of research into the aetiological importance of the social environment and the epidemiology of psychiatric disorders, the reader is referred to the report of the Milbank Memorial Conference in 1952 (567).

Commenting on recent research trends, Ahrenfeldt remarked in a working paper that it is hardly necessary to emphasize the fact that there remains an immense unexplored field of mental health problems requiring further study: e.g. vulnerable states in the life cycle; human relationship formation in various cultures; factors promoting stability and psychological strength in various cultures. He also drew attention to the need for initiative to be taken now in mental health research in relation to the exploration of outer space, including study of those who conceive and plan interplanetary excursions and cosmic conquests, and of the selection and training of personnel.

In anticipation of Ahrenfeldt's comment, the Scientific Committee of WFMH published in 1961 a cross-cultural study on Mental Health and Value Systems (41), which opened an inquiry into the compatibility of contemporary mental health concepts with various religions and ideologies. Among many further research areas suggested by this study, the following appear to be the most significant: processes by which the child becomes oriented; the development of communication systems, and the effects of interruption of relationships; the definiteness or otherwise of social role, and the relationships of individual aspiration to community goals; different ways of introducing mental health work in various communities; the differentiation of the various functions of professional people; attitudes towards mental illness; growth, change, and maturity; identity-formation; intensity of emotional relationships; responsibility and authority.

DIAGNOSTIC TECHNIQUES AND THERAPEUTIC METHODS
We have discussed above (p. 45) some aspects of the present chaos in the fields of diagnosis and of psychiatric nomenclature, and have noted that there has been little appreciable improvement either in techniques or in the accuracy of scientific diagnosis in recent years. There is, therefore, a most urgent need for further research and studies in these areas. Among recent valuable contributions in this field we would mention a survey of the uses and predictive limitations of intelligence tests in infants and young children (440); a number of follow-up and prediction studies of juvenile delinquents (321, 472, 552); and a follow-up study by Ginzberg et al. (137) of the military history and subsequent adjustment to civilian life of servicemen in the United States after World War II.

The view was expressed in the Study Group that the diagnostic techniques used in psychiatry have reached the end of a particular developmental phase; that it is now widely accepted that present psychiatric techniques are inadequate as the sole means of recognizing impending or early mental dysfunction or social maladjustment. This applies both in respect of individuals and in respect of the community, in different, and for the most part unexplored, cultural environments. The Study Group was in agreement that research in this area should carry a very high priority, particularly in relation to the social and cultural factors involved. There are three main directions:

(a) Investigations that might lead towards a better capacity to identify gradually developing symptoms of deviant individual and social behaviour (see also Volume II, Chapter 7). A major objective would be the establishment of a series of indicators, possibly of widespread significance and applicability, of imminent or early individual or social breakdown, to include the rationalization of local knowledge and suppositions about particular illnesses. As a longer-term aim, the eduction of principles on which to base wider developments of case-finding practices is highly important.

(b) Parallel to (a) is improvement of the case-finding training of professional personnel and of the case-finding education of the public. This involves working out and introducing methods of professional training and public (including parental) education that are appropriate to specific cultures, in order to develop the sensibilities necessary for a better understanding of the significance of mental health problems. It would be a specific aim to foster the ability to recognize, with a reasonable degree of accuracy, early forms of mental maladjustment and incipient breakdown, particularly among children. We should also search for better ways of introducing mental health principles into existing public health practice, which Lin (97) regards as essentially a matter of education. The study of methods of training teachers, throughout the whole range of the educational system, to enable them to recognize which are the real 'problem children' who are in need of treatment, is another task of high priority. We need to be able to distinguish, at an early stage, between those children who should be given psychological treatment and those who, though they may show more obvious and disturbing behaviour disorders, would benefit more from a good education (in the widest sense), given by teachers with a sound mental health training and deep psychological insight, than from psychotherapy.

(c) Study of the effects of different social environments, and, in particular, of sudden and marked changes in the environment, on the behaviour and adaptability of unstable and deviant individuals.

In a reference to the diagnostic methods now in use in mental health work, Skard remarked in a working paper that many of the techniques, especially projective testing, have been developed on the basis of clinical work with problem children and proceed by hypotheses that are also formed from clinical experience. She advocated the testing-out of diagnostic instruments on a wider range including a representative number of presumably normal children, and also the repeating of investigations in different cultures. Skard wrote:

'For such methods as, for example, the World Test, it is not enough to have a rich experience in problem children. It would also be advantageous to have, as a frame of reference, data from normal children of different ages in various cultures. The same might be said about other projective tests, such as the TAT and similar picture tests (e.g. W. Henry *et al.*), and Frustration Tests (e.g. the Lerner Blocking Techniques, the Rosenzweig P.F. tests). Studies of these kinds would not only provide a better basis for judging what is "normal" and to what extent a certain child may be deviating from the normal at a certain age. They would also furnish valuable data for the comparison of child development in different cultures, and on similarities and differences from one group of children to another. Much research is still needed in this area.'

There was support in the Study Group for the view that, on the whole, personality assessment techniques are unsatisfactory at present, even for use strictly within a particular culture, and that they have not reached a level of refinement that makes them useful to any extent across cultural boundaries. This does not mean that they are not capable of being applicable in trans-cultural contexts, but that this is a field in which much basic research is still needed. The Study Group accepted the view that serious errors leading to misdiagnosis are being made in the interpretation of results, especially in the case of young children, because insufficient allowance has been made for the fact that nearly all tests have a high cultural specificity. It is essential to ensure that all psychological tests (intelligence, personality, aptitude, attainment, etc.) are culturally appropriate to the test subject.

It is desirable to improve not only the psychological tests in use but also, and this may be even more important, the interview setting within which such tests are normally given. Skard wrote in a working paper:

'Beside the tests (developmental and projective) the *interview* is an important instrument in all clinical psychological and psychiatric work. The *anamnesis or history-taking* furnishes a picture of the past of the patient as seen by himself or by relatives (parents, etc.). We may regard the information obtained in this way both as an expression of the mind of the interviewed person at the time when he is being interviewed and as facts about the past. In the latter case, how reliable is the information obtained? As part of our investigation of our eighteen cases, the mothers were asked after seven or eight years about data already known to us from information gained earlier. Reliability varied much from individual to individual, and we were unable to tell from other cues which individuals would "tell the truth". Also, reliability varied according to the nature of the questions, information about such facts as weight at birth, etc. being much more reliable than information about emotions and attitudes.

'However, this is only one aspect of the problem. It would also be important to know which data and episodes the interviewed person brings out easily, and which are forgotten or not spontaneously remembered at the time of the interview. It would be of great interest to have this problem investigated within a longitudinal study where data were available for purposes of control at each stage of the children's development.

'Much research work is needed in the whole field of mental hygiene, and the problems mentioned above are only a few instances. It remains very important to redouble our efforts to study not only the development and personality formation of normal children but also deviation from normal development and its causes.'

On the clinical side, the Study Group thought that there is now a general measure of agreement that the existence of a more or less unbridged gap between those who are concerned with better understanding of the physiology and biochemistry of the brain and those who study behaviour and psychodynamics has seriously delayed progress in psychiatry. There is a great need for research projects to bridge the gap, and it was noted with satisfaction that research on mental illness nowadays has been increasingly concerned with chemical, psychobiological, and social factors, respectively, in more equal proportions. The two main factors limiting research in these fields at present are money, especially for long-term support, and the lack of available experienced research personnel. As we have remarked above, one of the more serious difficulties of doing original work in this field is that, whereas so much research into mental health, illness, and disorder is necessarily exploratory in character, very often its value and worthiness for support are judged by people with little first-hand experience of mental health research techniques, and especially of interdisciplinary work.

In the field of therapy there have been two main growing-points in research since 1948: (i) study of the effects and side-effects of the ataractic and psychotropic drugs, and their application to clinical psychiatry (215, 222, 224, 236); and (ii) study of various aspects of psychotherapy in relation to different social and cultural environments (213, 386). Widespread activity in these therapeutic fields is of such recent development, and has grown so rapidly in depth and intensity, that it must be conceded that techniques have generally outstripped rationale, so that the need for comprehensive research is great.

There have been a number of independent investigations in various countries concerning the factors influencing length of stay in mental hospitals, and the discharge and subsequent adjustment of chronic psychiatric patients. These studies are, however, of limited and local significance, and we have heard of no attempt at a coordinated investigation of this kind, at a national level, from which 'discharge prediction' techniques might be derived. Kramer (110) points out that:

'Accurate follow-up data on discharged mental patients can serve as the basis for "discharge prediction" techniques, weighting significant factors in the patient's life history, diagnosis, clinical course in hospital, degree of improvement, and expected family and community environment. Furthermore, better understanding of relapse factors would greatly aid the development of rehabilitation programmes for patients, while they are still in the hospital and later when they have returned to the community.'

In an experimental study with a transcultural involvement, WFMH US Committee, Inc., with the support of the Office of Vocational Rehabilitation, US Department of Health, Education, and Welfare, investigated some aspects of the vocational rehabilitation of discharged mental hospital patients in two areas of the United States (Delaware and Hawaii) and of England (Cambridgeshire and Essex). By means of questionnaires, inquiries have been carried out into the attitudes of professional staffs of mental hospitals towards the rehabilitation aspects of their work, and into the attitudes of key persons in the community towards the rehabilitation of discharged mental hospital patients (A. R. Askenasy and M. Zavalloni, 1963). A further small inquiry has been initiated into the experiences of the ex-patients themselves. It is hoped that this project will provide valuable material for further studies in this field.

The Study Group also considered some aspects of action research, in addition to the more basic projects that have been discussed. A particularly practical field of study concerns the provision of emergency social, medical, and psychiatric services for use in countries where facilities are non-existent. One suggestion advocated a carefully controlled study to evaluate the results of setting up small welfare groups in local communities, whose members could be alerted to individual problems arising in the mental health field from sickness, depression, and so on, and who would have had training to enable them to give a 'first-aid' kind of help. The major social advantage of this suggestion is that ordinary people in the community would become personally involved in health work. The Study Group recognized that it might be very difficult to bring this proposal into effective operation because of questions of confidence and the unwillingness of people to allow their problems to become common property – and this is why it is being advanced as a matter for active research rather than as immediate policy.

EPIDEMIOLOGICAL STUDIES
A recent growing-point, internationally, of research in the mental health field has been the application of methods of preventive medicine research to mental health problems. The techniques developed for the study of communicable diseases have been found remarkably useful in studies of the distribution of the major mental illnesses, and the epidemiology of mental disorder is rapidly becoming a subject in its own right. It is true that this subject is still in its infancy, but the WHO Expert Committee on Mental Health (129) has put forward suggestions about research, and a number of other valuable papers have appeared (104, 109, 111, 115, 116, 120, 128). WHO convened an interregional conference at Naples in 1960 to discuss techniques of conducting surveys on the epidemiology of mental disorder, and included participants from other than European and North American countries (130).

The need for much more comparative study in this field is universally agreed, to include the incidence and prevalence of mental disorders in different cultures, and the ecological, ethological, and cultural factors that may be of aetiological significance. At present, the usefulness of such studies for cross-cultural comparison is severely limited by the lack of a generally acceptable and uniform nomenclature of mental disorders (59). Some of the problems that arise in epidemiological studies are well illustrated in a paper by Tizard (363) on the prevalence of mental subnormality.

As one of many possible examples of the urgent need for more study in this field, we may cite the lack of statistically valid data on the number of emotionally ill children requiring inpatient treatment – a lack that makes it impossible to estimate on any other basis than a guess the required number of beds for this purpose in any given area (281).

The Study Group considered that the application of epidemiological method should not be restricted to mental disorders, but could be profitably introduced over a wider field of health promotion and prophylactic action. But whatever the field, and although most informed people are in full agreement that there is a need for vastly improved and more numerous survey projects, it may be felt that under current conditions this recommendation is little more than an expression of pious hope. The techniques of medical epidemiology are notoriously difficult to acquire, and considerable periods of training and experience are necessary in order to gain proficiency. There is no field of epidemiological study so little explored, where the social factors are so complex and where so few competent professional people have been operating, as that of mental health and disorder. It is clear that if work in this area is left in the hands of professional people alone, for numerical reasons no great volume of achievement can be expected within the next professional generation.

The question was put, therefore, whether more progress might be gained through less ambitious survey projects, perhaps undertaken by non-professional people working under the guidance of experts. To some it may appear very wasteful that so little concerted effort is being made to use the vast clinical experience now being obtained in the field of mental health and disorder for the further organization of aetiological and psychopathological knowledge.

Interest has recently centred on the possibility of making up what might be referred to as a 'do-it-yourself' kit, in order to gain epidemiological information. In essentials, this is a set of procedures – questionnaires, sampling devices, and so on – that might be placed in the hands of more or less untrained people in order to elicit certain kinds of information in a given community. This idea has been put forward in full recognition that it would be by no means a simple operation. Not only are there immense emotionally based difficulties to be anticipated in the getting of reliable information from untrained people about mental illness and behaviour disorders in their own families and communities; but also the sheer difficulty of knowing what to look for and how to interpret evidence when it is obtained is not a little daunting at the outset.

A psychiatrist remarked that, following a suggestion made at a WHO meeting on epidemiology that such do-it-yourself kits might be developed, it had been calculated that preparation of the instrument might occupy perhaps as long as one and a half years, and a further year would be required to refine it in a series of pilot schemes; an additional year would then be spent checking the kit on selected samples in various parts of the world. Thus it would be at least three and a half years before the kit could be published, and its cost might well amount to $50,000. It would be, therefore, both costly and time-consuming, as was the WHO publication on the epidemiology of mental disorder (120), which took about three years to produce and involved a number of small international, cross-disciplinary conferences.

The United States Joint Commission on Mental Illness and Health (389), in response to a considerable demand, encouraged experimentally the conduct of small surveys by communities about to plan new mental health provisions, the communities doing the work themselves with their own resources. This initiative resulted in the publication of a so-called Orange Book, compiled by a group of sociologists, social psychologists, psychologists, and so on. It had been originally intended to get experts to compile a handbook first, and then to encourage communities to study it before asking a consultant to help them to plan, but in fact many communities got to work on their own. Some of the larger cities made quite sophisticated surveys, but on the whole the smaller rural communities worked more by rule of thumb. It was generally thought that a great deal of good came out of these activities, not only in the provision of more appropriate facilities, but also in the involvement of the local people themselves. It was considered, however, by the Joint Commission that the Orange Book had only a very specific use within the boundaries of the United States (for which it was written) and that its direct application to other parts of the world should be discouraged.

The Study Group concluded from this discussion that the compilation of do-it-yourself kits for general use is practicable only region by region and within relatively narrow limits. A psychiatrist with experience of these matters in the Caribbean area was of the opinion that it would be possible, for example, to produce a survey kit to serve a number of contiguous islands, without necessarily producing separate kits for each island. However, although the specificity of the actual kits may be conceded, this does not mean that it may not be very useful to draw up some general principles on the basis of which particular survey projects could be considered.

The Study Group noted the warning of one of its psychiatrist members most experienced in epidemiological studies that it could be unfortunate to stir up any widespread interest in the possibility that major surveys might be undertaken by such do-it-yourself methods, by people without advanced scientific training in this field. However urgent it may be to learn more about the epidemiology of mental disorders, these do-it-yourself projects must be kept at a very simple level of information-collecting if they are not to incur the danger of leading to entirely misleading interpretations, based on incomplete and possibly inaccurate data.

A major motive of the Study Group in advocating an immediate increase of survey activity even by limited do-it-yourself techniques is that, in an era of easy communications and rapid social and cultural evolution, potentially useful opportunities for research are being lost almost every day as traditional ways of life give way before so-called progress and development. Because of the relative simplicity of the field of study much has been learnt from the analysis of patterns of social behaviour in more isolated communities, but all over the world such isolation is disappearing.

For example, in a remote area of the south-east of the Sudan, the normal life of the boys of a certain tribe includes an institutionalized homosexual phase. A study of this interesting social phenomenon has been undertaken, and this will be the last opportunity for doing it, for it is quite clear that as the communications of the country open up this particular tribal custom will not survive. Apparently it is the usual practice in this tribe for adult men to 'sponsor' a prepubertal boy with whom they form an affective relationship. This is accepted as normal in the community. The follow-up study has shown that whereas the majority of these boys, towards the end of adolescence, establish normal heterosexual relationships, a minority continue in a homosexual pattern.

The investigation is producing evidence to suggest that those boys who later become normal have passed through the homosexual phase mainly in response to environmental pressure with little constitutional involvement; even in those who continue in a passive type of homosexuality the constitutional influence appears to have been only slight; but more active persistent homosexuality appears to have a more definitely mixed constitutional and environmental aetiology. The psychological typology of the adult sponsors is not yet known, but it would be interesting if, in due course, the logical induction is confirmed that sponsors are found among those who, after their own experience of being sponsored as boys, remain as persistent active homosexuals.

This Sudanese tribe offers a good example of an experimental situation already set up by circumstances and facilitating the study of a particular phenomenon in a relatively uncomplicated setting. Simple survey methods and do-it-yourself kits could be of great assistance in the identification of other possible experimental situations, which might then be studied before they disappear in processes of cultural change. This is a major reason to act without further delay, even by relatively simple means, rather than wait until more truly scientific inquiries can be organized.

RESPONSIBILITY FOR THE PROMOTION OF RESEARCH

In their report, Krapf and Moser (5) noted a tendency in several countries for government-financed institutes to be set up for research in the mental health field, in some cases solely in this field and in others as part of government medical research institutes on a wider plane. Mention of government research institutes was made by thirteen countries responding to their inquiry. We welcome the evidence of an increasing governmental sense of responsibility for the encouragement and support of research projects, but we would not wish to minimize the danger, in some parts of the world, of scientific work in this field coming too directly under political influences. This warning brings us to the verge of a wide social problem of current concern, which is outside the range of this part of our discussions but which we have discussed at length in Volume II (Chapter 6). It is that of the role of the scientist as a citizen, and the moral aspects of his relationship with his own community and the world.

The Study Group discussed the varied and often naïve attitudes of governments to the role of the scientist and to research, and the tendency to create new institutions by legislation without a serious attempt to find out where the activity is likely to lead, and without provision for the evaluation of results. In a working paper referring primarily to the United Kingdom, Fox commented:

'It is a peculiar fact of governmental action – in the UK at any rate – that millions may be voted to welfare services of different kinds without any thought of finding out whether the money is being well spent. The *Penal system* offers probation services, attendance centres, detention centres, approved schools, borstals and various kinds of prison and after-care with no idea if any of them work, or of what sorts of effects what kinds of penal treatment have on which varieties of

offender. The *National Assistance Board* offers relief to desti-
tute and handicapped people but there is still no planned
effort to discover the origins of problem families or to reduce
the chronic invalidism of accident neurosis, or unemploy-
ability due to different kinds of handicap. The *Education Acts*
have set up a vast national system of graded schools and entry
thereto by an examination at 11+, but without any planned
intention to see if it turns out well.

'A welcome and, I believe, unique departure was the UK
Ministry of Health's recent announcement on proposed centres
for the classification and treatment of psychopaths. Due partly
to the prompting of a Medical Research Council sub-committee
on psychopaths which met at the same time as the Ministry's
working party, research was written in from the outset,
related both to the psychopath himself and to the effects upon
him of the treatment process.'

It would seem to be no more than prudent conduct, whenever
social legislation is contemplated, to make provision in the legislation for evaluation and scientific control from the outset, and
for a continuous programme of research into ways of improving
techniques and methods. It is important to ensure not only that
public effort and money are being well spent, but also that
research and evaluation become an integral part of social action;
that the latter should no longer be regarded as an outside or
luxury activity dependent on charitable Foundations or the part-
time services of a few interested scientists, with all the arbitrari-
ness and lack of coordination that are likely to arise when it is so
regarded.

THE RESEARCH ROLE OF WFMH

The question of how an international non-governmental organization like the WFMH can contribute to research activity is
complex. It is a truism to point out that research activity in the
human sciences cannot easily be divorced from a particular
location, and therefore the practical research function of an
international organization may be difficult to establish con-

vincingly. In general, the Study Group thought that the most appropriate role of WFMH would be in the triple function of facilitating comparative studies, exchange of personnel, and the dissemination of research information where it is most needed.

As an example of the facilitation of comparative studies we have already discussed a contribution that WFMH might make by sponsoring the preparation of a series of guides for the making of operational research observations. These would embody descriptions of various existing projects, the lesson that had been learnt from them, and any warnings that could be given on a basis of past experience. They might include suggestions about what the individual professional worker might look out for in the normal course of duty that could be of use to others working and making inquiries in the field. A possible by-product of such guides could be the preparation of manuals in simple terms offering a kind of distillate of the experience of clinical workers for the use of people concerned with school and family counselling, and like activities.

A particularly useful and appropriate role for WFMH, in the opinion of some members of the Study Group, is to assume responsibility for the distribution of available funds to those individuals and institutions with whom and where they would have the greatest effect. These members thought that, while the actual promotion of operational research, particularly of an epidemiological type, can be undertaken effectively by intergovernmental organizations, these latter are not so well placed to give advice to independent fund-granting organizations about the expenditure of research funds.

The essential functions of critical appraisal of existing mental health work, and assessment of need and opportunity, can very well be undertaken by governmental and non-governmental organizations in combination. The Study Group was of the opinion that the role of WFMH as a consultant to WHO and other UN specialized agencies could be developed with advantage to a greater extent than has been the case up to now. WFMH has a relatively high degree of organization through its network of membership in forty-four countries, and it could be of the greatest possible assistance to the UN agencies, provided that the latter are able to make full use of such help, in furnishing information about personnel, opportunities, and needs, and in supplementing or complementing official action. This appears to be one of the most effective ways in which private citizens with specialist qualifications can contribute effectively to international work at this level.

The best role of WFMH as a research instrument was very well described in a working paper by Fox:

'The primary usefulness of an international mental health organization such as the World Federation for Mental Health is, to my mind, the encouragement, sponsorship or financing, of useful research efforts in many places. Not only are these of interest in themselves and of importance to the country concerned for planning purposes, but the international correlation of differences in mental and social illness with differences in social structure, may offer valuable clues to the origins of disorder. It follows therefore that studies in different places might give most benefit if they were co-ordinated centrally, and made to measure the same thing at the same time. E.g. suicide – its incidence and distribution by social class, age, sex, occupation, time of day, place of residence – per Durkheim and his followers (E. Durkheim, *Suicide* (1897)). Such subjects must be fairly simply definable, detectable, and susceptible to study without elaborate equipment and highly sophisticated or untried techniques.

'While effort in other fields may be of value, teaching, prevention and propaganda efforts are hampered by lack of facts and agreed definitions, and are more open to destructive scientific and political criticisms. Also I hold them of less value at the present state of knowledge. But tributes to research are regularly paid by everyone – lip-service and otherwise – and people of different cultures and faiths could probably unite in the search for knowledge more readily than in most things.'

In order to fulfil an advisory role effectively, however, international non-governmental organizations must be so placed that they command the respect both of individual scientists and institutions and of governments. This is best ensured by the personal records of the individuals employed by the voluntary organization on advisory duties. They need to have personal experience of successful interdisciplinary and transcultural research activities. The advisory role of the voluntary organization is greatly strengthened when it has itself a record of making original contributions to knowledge in some cognate field.

THE CLEARING-HOUSE FUNCTION

The Study Group was convinced that improvement of the current information services about research would greatly benefit future research activity. In no country is there an organization able, effectively and comprehensively, to coordinate information about existing research projects in the wide field of the human sciences. This would be, of course, an undertaking of immense magnitude; and in view of the complications of language and distance, it may well be practical to think in terms of the establishment of a number of regional clearing-houses of information rather than of a single universal one.

There was some division of opinion in the Study Group as to the relative merits of the clearing-house type of proposal, on the one hand, and the less highly organized but more direct method of dissemination of information by the convening of international, interdisciplinary conferences for the exchange of information and the discussion of new ideas, on the other.

The outstanding example of the successful performance of the clearing-house function is that of the Bio-Sciences Information Exchange of the Smithsonian Institute in Washington. The principal objective here is to list every research project in the field of biological science, anywhere in the world, that is in receipt of financial support from the United States Public Health Service, other US governmental sources, or a Foundation in the United States. In addition, those responsible for other research activities in any part of the world not enumerated among the above are invited to contribute full information about their work for inclusion in the list. The Bio-Sciences Exchange, as the name implies, is concerned only incidentally with projects in the mental health field among very many other fields, but in order to give an impression of the size of this vast undertaking – admittedly incomplete though it may be – we might add that, in the section on mental health projects, 1957–58, we counted more than 2,000 mental health research projects undertaken by nearly 500 institutions dispersed throughout the United States. We were given to understand that this probably represented the great bulk of mental health research projects in existence in the United States at that time. Inspection showed that the research projects listed were very largely, though not entirely, limited to work in the fields of clinical psychiatry, experimental psychology, neurology, and neurophysiology. There were relatively few projects concerned with the wider, and in our view more immediately rewarding, interdisciplinary and preventive aspects of mental health.

In a working paper Ahrenfeldt commented that the titles of the projects listed in the Bio-Sciences Information Exchange indicate the comparatively high popularity among research workers in the mental health field of observational studies on the behaviour of experimental animals. He remarked that some of the titles give food for thought about the way in which research workers are currently conceptualizing their task. No doubt the titles of research projects may be an imprecise, even unreliable, guide to the researchers' actual intentions, but they do, presumably, embody what the applicants think will appeal to the fund-granting agency. As we have discussed earlier in this chapter, in these days of the centralization of research money in the hands of a comparatively few governmental and non-governmental fund-granting agencies, a study of the titles and the scope of the research projects that have been successful in gaining financial support is a useful indication of trends.

Ahrenfeldt asked what could legitimately be said about titles like the two following examples, taken at random from many similar ones: (i) 'Evaluation of concepts of learning, homeostasis, and palatability' (in the text the project was explained further: 'Rats, chickens, and humans will be given various behavioural tests for different sugars . . . etc.'). (ii) 'The effects of group living versus isolation on hyperphagia in rats with electrolytic lesions of the anterior medial hypothalmic nuclei' ('the effects of group living on this behaviour will be explored'). In our view, these titles show evidence of unclear concept-formation. In the former title, three dissimilar and heterogeneous abstract concepts are grouped together for study, by administering different sugars to three unrelated natural orders of animals which have non-comparable styles of social organization. Very strong methodological objections might be lodged both against the presence of so many variable and uncontrolled factors in a single experiment, and against the attempt to extrapolate the data for the elucidation of three such complex abstract concepts. With regard to the second title one might question the validity of extrapolation to spontaneous animal behaviour any conclusions drawn from observations of the behaviour of animals in captivity, and of comparing behaviour in an artificially determined group with behaviour in equally artificially determined isolation after a mutilating injury, the precise extent of which cannot be finely controlled, has been inflicted on the animals concerned.

How far these two projects indicate any more widespread attitude could be judged only by a comprehensive survey of research schemes wherever they may be found. The above examples emphasize the importance of finding out precisely what is going on in this field, but the experience of the Washington Bio-Sciences Exchange illustrates the extreme costliness of the attempt, in money and in personnel time. The Bio-Sciences Exchange is in a class of its own; in no other place is there a source of information about projects that even approaches this one for completeness, and in most places there is not even a rudimentary basis from which to start. But the Exchange is only incidentally concerned with mental health and aims to be comprehensive only in regard to the United States.

There is no general conviction that the usefulness of indexes and information exchanges at a world level can justify the astronomical expense of keeping them exhaustive and up to date. Acting on a suggestion originally made by UNESCO, WFMH has been seeking for some years to establish an index of mental health projects, with the ultimate objective of providing a world-wide coverage, but not necessarily by the establishment of a single information-dispensing institute. In fact, it is more likely that if this scheme comes to fruition the great bulk of the work will be done through the cooperation of existing centres in various regions. It has proved extremely difficult to find even modest support for this plan, but at the time of writing (1964) WFMH, under contract with the United States National Institute of Health, has set up a small pilot project in Geneva on the collection of research information in Europe, with a view to the progressive development of more comprehensive information services.

The Study Group noted with appreciation the efforts of a number of individuals to promote an exchange in certain selected fields of interest, and, in particular, the *Review* and *Newsletter* on transcultural research in mental health problems, published by the Section of Transcultural Psychiatric Studies of the Department of Psychiatry, McGill University, Montreal, and concerned with cross-cultural studies of a more anthropological nature; and journal-abstracting services inaugurated in the universities of Santiago de Chile and Heidelberg. Such individual efforts, however, are severely restricted by the prohibitive cost of setting up an effective network of information collection, without which the gaining of information must necessarily be largely fortuitous, being based on the personal contacts of a relatively few people.

As an alternative to the clearing-house idea there is the possibility, discussed above, of holding series of international, inter-disciplinary, and transnational working conferences. This method of disseminating information is in no way in opposition to the clearing-house function; indeed, the two proposals are complementary. One member of the Study Group estimated that the amount of money necessary to maintain an adequate international register of mental health research might finance perhaps forty international conferences in a year, and it may be arguable that the spread of information from the conferences would be much wider than it could possibly be from a register.

The Study Group was in no doubt that the small interdisciplinary conference is one of the best ways of achieving depth of discussion, and of trying out new ideas; that it can perform an evaluation function and stimulate new work in ways that are quite unlikely to result from any scheme for a register. The work of a conference, however, is more ephemeral than that of a register, and likely to be influenced more by passing modes of thought. The Study Group agreed that both registers and conferences are highly desirable, and it deprecated reports that it is becoming more difficult to get financial support for interdisciplinary discussion groups. The members have noted with great regret the discontinuance of the justly famed Macy Conferences and the work of the Psychobiological Group of WHO, and, nearer to the heart of WFMH itself, the disbandment of the Scientific Committee of WFMH and the discontinuance of the series of cross-national interdisciplinary reports – owing to lack of financial support. There appears to be no comparable initiative in the international mental health field at present that may compensate for the loss of these institutions.

The question of an international institute of mental health, which has long been a dream of WFMH, was little discussed in the Study Group, mainly because the concept of an institute did not appear to be highly practicable under current conditions. There is support for the view that mental health investigations and studies can best be done in the field by local people; that the gathering together of experienced scientists in a central organization may prove to be an expensive embarrassment rather than a real aid to good work; and that it is more practical to set up regional institutes of modest size as service stations for fieldwork teams in regions of not too great cultural diversity. Such service stations would be mainly concerned with facilitating field teams, and giving expert consultative help on experimental design, statistical method and operations, and the like.

SOME SUGGESTED FIELDS OF WORK

Without attempting to be exhaustive, the Study Group discussed a few suggestions for mental health research activities that, it was thought, might give immediate and significant results.

Studies of Success in Research

It was proposed to examine the history and development of a number of mental health research projects which were recognized to have had an outstanding success and in which something really notable had happened. A careful historical compilation of the sequence of events that had led to the result in each case might help towards the understanding of what makes for success in mental health research. In this way it might be possible to test the perhaps complacent notion of natural scientists that the sequence of events that leads to success in research in this field is entirely a matter of logical reasoning. It may legitimately be wondered whether, in those cases where the creative impulse of the individual research worker does not fall into any of the fields currently accorded a high priority, or follow the methods now orthodox for the natural sciences, there is a danger that much valuable research impetus may be lost.

Immediate Action

One very fruitful way of promoting mental health research might be to concentrate on those cross-cultural or transnational research projects that could be started immediately, and for which the necessary technical knowledge and equipment are already available. Such projects would, by definition, be limited and would not require highly sophisticated resources. The criteria of priority would be based more on feasibility than on urgency. It would be valuable for WFMH to sponsor an international group to examine, advise on, and recommend projects for immediate adoption.

Studies of Change

In Volume II we have made several references to the desirability of studying various cultural phenomena in areas of rapid change, before such phenomena vanish. This suggestion refers broadly to a programme of research rather than to definite projects, and might be applicable almost anywhere in the world. One specific proposal, which might pass the test of feasibility, is to select a previously stable rural community, which is at an early stage in the processes of urbanization or other major social change, and make a detailed record of all instances that can be found of effective traditional methods of handling the mentally ill or subnormal. The records could be used, not so much as a baseline from which to enter upon new social advances, but as information about the principles of social care most suited to that community. For this purpose it would be necessary to analyse what it was in the previous circumstances that made the method effective, and how the method could be applied to the changing conditions of that society.

Attitudes to Illness

A recurrent theme in our discussions has been our need to know more about various cultural attitudes to the mentally ill and to psychological illness, to behaviour disturbances, and to the impact of social change. We have advocated the permeation of such studies by more modern epidemiological techniques. In this connexion the Study Group took note of the developing science of palaeopsychology, which is concerned with making comparative studies of the mentality of primitive people, of people at the lowest socio-economic levels of more advanced populations, and of the mental development of children. It is claimed that these studies are providing useful information about social change and development.

Use of Existing Personnel

The Study Group discussed a number of suggestions that local public health or social work personnel be used to collect

227

information about normal child-rearing practices and family behaviour patterns in given communities. A major difficulty about
such proposals is how best to set up the information-collecting
instruments for use by personnel at various levels and degrees of
scientific knowledge and sophistication. Further, much of the
information will have been collected and recorded in anecdotal
form, and is inevitably liable to distortion by the imposition of a
standard method of collection or recording. In spite of these real
difficulties it is considered that a great deal more could be
effected by such information-collecting methods than has been
attempted up to now.

We have already discussed this kind of proposal in the context
of do-it-yourself data-collecting kits – a term that is misleading
here because it wrongly implies the existence of ready-made
techniques and 'jigs' to get information. Although doubting the
practicability of such proposals in the present state of knowledge,
the Study Group agreed that every possible advantage should be
taken of the research potentialities of mental health workers, and
suggested that the Federation might consider how to give guidance about the effective collection of data. Although WFMH may
not currently be in a position to issue guides to information-
collecting in every mental health field, this suggestion is of considerable potential value and deserves further study.

Evaluation of Technical Assistance
Another practical suggestion of limited range in this area is that
WFMH should study the mental health aspects of selected UN and
other technical assistance programmes with a view to evaluation,
thus extending to these some of the sociological and economic
evaluations of technical assistance programmes that have been
undertaken by UNESCO.

Critical Periods in the Life-span
The Study Group thought that it would be valuable to delineate
for study certain critical periods in the individual life-history, and
institute more specific research programmes not only into the

phenomena of the critical period itself but also into the effects of such periods on the later life-history of the individual. The major critical periods are commonly listed as follows: birth, school entry, puberty and adolescence, school-leaving, work entry, marriage, entry into parenthood, the menopause, involution, retirement, and old age. We have noted above that whereas there has been a great deal of mental health work in connexion with children and young people, with women in the context of reproduction, and with old age, the whole period of early adulthood and middle age, particularly in the case of men, has been neglected. Subsequent to the International Study Group, the Scientific Committee adopted the topic of the mental health of men in the forty to sixty age group as its third cross-cultural study.

Industrial Mental Health
Some members of the Study Group thought that there is a great need for study and research with a view to the publication of handbooks on mental health principles for industrial personnel workers, and that WFMH is well placed to sponsor their compilation. More specifically, the Study Group recommended the sponsoring of working conferences to inaugurate studies of work satisfaction in an automated society and of mental health aspects of such matters as rigid retirement-age rules and regulations.

Training in International Work
Lastly, earlier in this chapter we have discussed the use of transnational interdisciplinary conferences for the digestion of scientific information and its dissemination. Another type of conference procedure with rather different aims is that of the small international conference or colloquium which sets out to collect information concerning selected major mental health problems, and at the same time to serve as a training experience for young people in the field. This latter aim would be achieved by employing the younger workers on information-collecting and by having them sit in with the experts at the conference – a

procedure that the Scientific Committee of WFMH had hoped to adopt in connexion with its study of the mental health aspects of middle age. Unfortunately, as we have noted, it is proving very difficult to obtain financial support for these and similar promising leads, and this project had to be abandoned. This experience underlines the urgent need for new, courageous, and original thinking and planning in this whole field.

PART THREE

Bibliography

.

Bibliography

This bibliography has been compiled with the primary aim of including a significant proportion of the more important and representative publications that have appeared since 1948 in the very wide field of mental health, as well as such other works as have been referred to in the text.

In so vast a field there is necessarily, and fortunately, considerable overlap between subjects and disciplines, which has led to the adoption of a somewhat arbitrary method of classification, for purposes of presentation.

Each section of the bibliography is divided into two parts:

(i) Works identified by individual authors. Here items are arranged alphabetically under authors' names. Works by the same author are given in chronological order, and where there are two or more works by the same author in the same year these are listed alphabetically according to the first letter of the title.

(ii) Works of collective authorship. These publications (reports, studies, etc.) are listed alphabetically under the name of the organization concerned, the title of the work, or the country of origin, as may be appropriate. Where it is necessary, items are given in chronological order or alphabetically by title, as in (i) above.

Abbreviations of titles of periodicals are, in general, those of the *World List of Scientific Periodicals* (3rd edition, London, 1952).

In psychiatry and allied disciplines, the following periodical reviews of the literature will be found to be the most useful:

Monthly – *Excerpta medica, Amsterdam,* Section VIII (Neurology and Psychiatry).

BIBLIOGRAPHY

Annual – *Progress in Neurology and Psychiatry,* Ed. E. A. Spiegel, New York.

Annual – *Year Book of Neurology, Psychiatry and Neuro-surgery,* Present Eds. R. P. Mackay, S. B. Wortis & O. Sugar, Chicago.

In other branches of the human sciences concerned, reference should be made to the respective specialized periodicals and year-books which periodically review the literature in these fields.

CLASSIFICATION

235

The Field of Mental Health

MENTAL HEALTH PLANNING AND PERSPECTIVES

1 BROCKINGTON, F. (ed.) 1955. *Mental Health and the World Community*. WFMH, London.

2 DUBOS, R. 1959. *Mirage of Health: Utopias, Progress and Biological Change*. London.

3 KRAPF, E. E. 1959. 'The international approach to the problems of mental health.' *Int. soc. Sci. J.* 11: 63–71.

4 KRAPF, E. E. 1960. 'The work of the World Health Organization in the field of mental health.' *Ment. Hyg.* 44: 315–338.

5 KRAPF, E. E. & MOSER, J. 1962. 'Changes of emphasis and accomplishments in mental health work, 1948–1960.' *Ment. Hyg.* 46: 163–91. (Revised version of a working paper prepared for the Int. Study Group, Roffey Park, June 1961.)

6 LAIGNEL-LAVASTINE, M. & VINCHON, J. 1930. *Les Malades de l'esprit et leurs médecins du XVIe au XIXe siècle*. Paris. P. 14.

7 LEWIS, A. 1958. 'Between guesswork and certainty in psychiatry.' *Lancet* 1: 171–5, 227–30.

8 PATON, A. C. L. & KIDSON, M. C. (eds.) 1961. *First World Mental Health Year: A Record*. WFMH, London.

9 REES, J. R. 1958. 'The way ahead.' *Amer. J. Psychiat.* 115: 481–90.

10 SEMELAIGNE, R. 1930. *Les Pionniers de la psychiatrie française*. Tome 1. Paris.

11 THORNTON, E. M. (ed.) 1961. *Planning and Action for Mental Health* (12th & 13th Annual Meetings of WFMH – Barcelona, 1959 & Edinburgh, 1960). WFMH, London.

12 INTERNATIONAL PREPARATORY COMMISSION. 1948. *Mental Health and World Citizenship: A Statement prepared for the International Congress on Mental Health,*

London, 1948. WFMH, London. (English and German texts.)

13 WFMH. 1948. *Third International Congress on Mental Health, London, 1948.* Vol. 1: *History, Development and Organization*; Vol. 2: *Child Psychiatry*; Vol. 3: *Medical Psychotherapy*; Vol. 4: *Mental Hygiene.* 4 vols. WFMH, London.

14 WFMH. 1952. *Proceedings of the Fourth International Congress on Mental Health, Mexico City, 1951.* Mexico, D.F.

15 WFMH. 1954. *Mental Health in Public Affairs: A Report of the Fifth International Congress on Mental Health, Toronto, 1954.* Toronto.

16 WFMH. 1955. *Family Mental Health and the State* (8th Ann. Meeting WFMH, Istanbul, 1955). WFMH, London.

17 WFMH. 1956. *Bericht über die 6. Jahresversammlung der Weltvereinigung für Psychische Hygiene* (6th Ann. Meeting WFMH, Wien, 1953). Wien & Bonn.

18 WFMH. 1956. *Mental Health in Home and School* (9th Ann. Meeting WFMH, Berlin, 1956). WFMH, London.

19 WFMH. 1957. *Growing Up in a Changing World* (10th Ann. Meeting WFMH, Copenhagen, 1957). WFMH, London.

20 WFMH. 1960. *A Brief Record of Eleven Years, 1948–1959, and World Mental Health Year 1960.* WFMH, London.

21 WFMH. 1961. *Mental Health in International Perspective: A Review made in 1961 by an International and Interprofessional Study Group.* WFMH, London.

22 WFMH. 1961. *Proceedings of the VIth International Congress on Mental Health (Paris, 1961). Excerpta med. Int. Congr. Ser.* No. 45. Amsterdam.

23 WHO. 1950. Expert Committee on Mental Health: Report on the 1st Session. *World Hlth Org. tech. Rep. Ser.* 9. Geneva.

24 WHO. 1951. Expert Committee on Mental Health: Report on the 2nd Session. *World Hlth Org. tech. Rep. Ser.* 31. Geneva.

THE CONCEPTUALIZATION OF MENTAL HEALTH

25 COBB, S. 1952. Foreword in *The Biology of Mental Health and Disease*. New York. Pp. xix–xxi.

26 DAVID, H. R. & BRENGELMANN, J. F. (eds.) 1960. *Perspectives in Personality Research*. London.

27 DICKS, H. V. 1959. *Mental Health in the light of Ancient Wisdom*. WFMH, London.

28 EL MAHI, T. 1960. 'Concept of mental health.' *E. Afr. med. J.* **37**: 472–6.

29 ERIKSON, E. H. 1956. 'The problem of ego identity.' *J. Amer. psychoanal. Ass.* **4**: 56–121.

30 GALDSTON, I. (ed.) 1960. *Human Nutrition, Historic and Scientific*. New York.

31 JAHODA, M. 1958. *Current Concepts of Positive Mental Health*. New York.

32 JUNG, C. G. 1958. *The Undiscovered Self* (transl. R. F. C. Hull). London.

33 KRAPF, E. E. 1961. 'The concepts of normality and mental health in psychoanalysis.' *Int. J. Psycho-Anal.* **42**: 439–46.

34 MASSERMAN, J. H. (ed.) 1959. *Individual and Familial Dynamics (Science and Psychoanalysis*, Vol. 2). New York. Part II: Familial and Social Dynamics. Pp. 90–214.

35 MASSERMAN, J. H. (ed.) 1960. *Psychoanalysis and Human Values (Science and Psychoanalysis*, Vol. 3). New York. Pp. 181–200.

36 MEAD, M. 1959. 'Mental health in world perspective.' In *Culture and Mental Health*, ed. M. K. Opler. New York. Pp. 501–16.

37 MEAD, M. 1962. 'Mental health and the wider world.' *Amer. J. Orthopsychiat.* **32**: 1–4.

38 RÜMKE, H. C. 1954. 'Solved and unsolved problems in mental health.' In *Mental Health in Public Affairs: A Report of the Fifth International Congress on Mental Health, Toronto*. Pp. 157 et seq.

39 SODDY, K. 1950. 'Mental health.' *Int. Hlth Bull. League of Red Cross Societies*, No. 2.

40 SODDY, K. (ed.) 1961. 'Identity.' In *Cross-cultural Studies in Mental Health*. London. Pp. 1–53. (First published as: *WFMH Introductory Study No. 1*, London, 1957.)

41 SODDY, K. (ed.) 1961. 'Mental health and value systems.' In *Cross-cultural Studies in Mental Health*. London. Pp. 55–261.

42 WHEELIS, A. 1958. *The Quest for Identity*. New York.

43 MILBANK MEMORIAL FUND. 1952. *The Biology of Mental Health and Disease* (27th Ann. Conf. Milbank Memorial Fund). New York.

44 PIUS XII. 1960. *Pie XII parle de santé mentale et de psychologie*. Bruxelles.

MENTAL HEALTH AND RELIGION

45 ANDERSON, G. C. 1956. 'Psychiatry's influence on religion.' *Pastoral Psychology*, Sept.

46 ANDERSON, G. C. 1960. *Current Conditions and Trends in Relations between Religion and Mental Health*. New York.

47 APPEL, K. E. *et al.* 1959. 'Religion.' In *American Handbook of Psychiatry*, ed. S. Arieti. New York. Vol. 2: 1777–810.

48 OATES, W. E. 1955. *Religious Factors in Mental Illness*. New York.

49 O'DOHERTY, E. F. 1956. 'Religion and mental health.' *Studies*, Spring. Dublin.

50 TILLICH, P. J. 1960. *The Impact of Psychotherapy on Theological Thought*. New York. (Also published in *Pastoral Psychology*, Feb. 1960.)

51 ACADEMY OF RELIGION AND MENTAL HEALTH. 1961. *Religion, Culture, and Mental Health* (Proc. 3rd Academy Symposium, Nov. 1959). New York.

PROBLEMS OF COMMUNICATION

52 CAPES, M. & WILSON, A. T. M. (eds.) 1960. *Communication or Conflict – Conferences: Their Nature, Dynamics, and Planning*. London.

53 CUNNINGHAM, J. M. 1952. 'Problems of communication in scientific and professional disciplines.' *Amer. J. Orthopsychiat.* **22**: 445–56.

54 EY, H. 1954. *Études psychiatriques.* Paris. Vol. 3: 32–45 (La Classification des maladies mentales).

55 FREMONT-SMITH, F. 1961. 'The interdisciplinary conference.' *Bull. Amer. Inst. biol. Sciences* **11**, No. 11 (Apr.): 17–20 & 32.

56 GLENN, E. S. 1954. 'Semantic difficulties in international communication.' *ETC: A Review of general Semantics* **11**: 163–80.

57 GLENN, E. S. *et al.* 1958. In *ETC: A Review of general Semantics* **15**: 81–151. Special issue on interpretation and intercultural communication (No. 2, Winter 1957–58).

58 RUESCH, J. 1958. 'Communication difficulties among psychiatrists.' In *Integrative Studies (Science and Psychoanalysis,* Vol. 1), ed. J. H. Masserman. New York. Pp. 85–100.

59 STENGEL, E. 1959. 'Classification of mental disorders.' *Bull. World Hlth. Org.* **21**: 601–63.

Clinical Aspects of Mental Health Action

REGIONAL QUESTIONS

60 ARIETI, S. (ed.) 1959. *American Handbook of Psychiatry.* 2 vols. New York.

61 BARTON, W. E. *et al.* 1961. *Impressions of European Psychiatry.* Amer. Psychiatr. Ass., Washington, D.C.

62 BELLAK, L. 1961. *Contemporary European Psychiatry.* New York.

63 CARAVEDO, B. 1959. 'Social psychiatry in Peru.' In *Progress in Psychotherapy*, eds. J. H. Masserman & J. L. Moreno. New York. Vol. 4: 321.

64 CASEY, J. F. & RACKOW, L. L. 1960. *Observations on the Treatment of the Mentally Ill in Europe.* Veterans Admin., Washington, D.C.

65 CHU, L. & LIU, M. 1960. 'Mental diseases in Peking between 1933 and 1943.' *J. ment. Sci.* **106**: 274–80.

66 DAVIES, S. P. 1960. *Toward Community Mental Health: A Review of the First Five Years of Operations under the Community Mental Health Services Act of the State of New York.* New York.

67 DUCHÊNE, H. 1959. *Les Services psychiatriques publics extra-hospitaliers* (Rapport au 57e Congrès de Psychiatrie et de Neurologie de langue française, Tours, 1959). Paris.

68 FIELD, M. G. 1960. 'Approaches to mental illness in Soviet society: some comparisons and conjectures.' *Social Problems* **7**: 277–97.

69 FORSTER, E. F. B. 1962. 'The theory and practice of psychiatry in Ghana.' *Amer. J. Psychother.* **16**: 7–51.

70 KLINE, N. S. 1960. *The Organization of Psychiatric Care and Psychiatric Research in the Union of Soviet Socialist Republics.* New York.

71 KRAPF, E. E. 1959. 'Les troubles mentaux des Africains et les problèmes de la psychiatrie comparée.' *Méd. et Hyg.*, *Genève*, **17**: 123–30.

72 LAMBO, T. A. 1955. 'The role of cultural factors in paranoid psychosis among the Yoruba tribe (Nigeria).' *J. ment. Sci.* **101**: 239–66.

73 LAMBO, T. A. 1956. 'Neuropsychiatric observations in the Western Region of Nigeria.' *Brit. med. J.* **2**: 1388–94.

74 LAMBO, T. A. 1959. 'Mental health in Nigeria.' *World ment. Hlth.* **11**: 131–8. (Reprinted, ibid., 1961, **13**: 135–41.)

75 LAMBO, T. A. 1960. 'Further neuropsychiatric observations in Nigeria, with comments on the need for epidemiological study in Africa.' *Brit. med. J.* **2**: 1696–704.

76 LAMBO, T. A. 1960. 'The concept and practice of mental health in African cultures.' *E. Afr. med. J.* **37**: 464–71.

77 MARGETTS, E. L. 1960. 'The future for psychiatry in East Africa.' *E. Afr. med. J.* **37**: 448–56.

78 MORA, G. 1959. 'Recent American psychiatric developments.' In *American Handbook of Psychiatry*, ed. S. Arieti. New York. Vol. 1: 20–21.

79 PACHECO E SILVA, A. C. 1960. 'Mental hygiene in underdeveloped countries.' *World ment. Hlth* **12**: 18–23.

80 PATERSON, A. S. 1959. 'The practice of psychiatry in England under the National Health Service, 1948–1959.' *Amer. J. Psychiat.* **116**: 244–50.

81 SIVADON, P. 1958. 'Problèmes de santé mentale en Afrique noire.' *World ment. Hlth* **10**: 106–19.

82 SIVADON, P. 1959. 'Problèmes de santé mentale aux Caraïbes.' *World ment. Hlth* **11**: 122–30.

83 STOLLER, A. 1957. 'An Australian looks at the underdeveloped world.' In *Mental Health and the World Community*, ed. F. Brockington. WFMH, London. Pp. 31–9.

84 STRÖMGREN, E. 1958. 'Mental health service planning in Denmark.' *Danish med. Bull.***5**: 1–17.

85 TOOTH, G. 1950. *Studies in Mental Illness in the Gold Coast.* Colonial Res. Publ. No. 6. Colonial Office, London.

86 VYNCKE, J. 1957. 'Psychoses et névroses en Afrique centrale.' *Mém. Acad. R. Sci. colon.* Bruxelles, N.S., **5**: fasc. 5.

87 WORTIS, J. 1961. 'A psychiatric study tour of the USSR.' *J. ment. Sci.* **107**: 119–56.

88 CCTA/CSA. 1960. *Mental Disorders and Mental Health in Africa South of the Sahara (Bukavu, 1958).* Publ. No. 35. London.

89 *East African med. J.*, 1960. **37**: 443–85 (No. 6, June). Special Number: World Mental Health Year, 1960.

90 'The social problem of epilepsy in Peru.' 1960. *Amer. J. Psychiat.* **117**: 163–4.

91 WHO. 1959. *Seminar on Mental Health in Africa South of the Sahara (Brazzaville, 1958): Final Report.* WHO Regional Office for Africa, Brazzaville.

LOCAL PROGRAMMES

92 CARSE, J., PANTON, N. E. & WATT, A. 1958. 'A district mental health service: The Worthing experiment.' *Lancet* **1**: 39–41.

93 COLEMAN, M. D. & ZWERLING, I. 1959. 'The psychiatric emergency clinic: A flexible way of meeting mental health needs.' *Amer. J. Psychiat.* **115**: 980–4.

94 FREEMAN, H. L. 1960. 'Oldham and District psychiatric service.' *Lancet* **1**: 218–21.

95 LEMKAU, P. V. & CROCETTI, G. M. 1961. 'The Amsterdam municipal psychiatric service: A psychiatric-sociological review.' *Amer. J. Psychiat.* **117**: 779–83.

96 LEYBERG, J. T. 1959. 'A district psychiatric service: The Bolton pattern.' *Lancet* **2**: 282–4.

97 LIN, T. 1961. 'Evolution of mental health programmes in Taiwan.' *Amer. J. Psychiat.* **117**: 961–71.

98 QUERIDO, A. 1954. 'Domiciliary psychiatry: The Amsterdam experiment.' *Brit. med. J.* **2**: 1043.

99 QUERIDO, A. 1956. 'Early diagnosis and treatment services.' In *The Elements of a Community Mental Health Program.* Milbank Memorial Fund, New York. Pp. 158–181.

100 EDINBURGH CORPORATION. 1959. *Mental Health Services – Edinburgh: A Plan for Co-ordinated Development.* Report by a Medical Working Party. Edinburgh.

101 NEW YORK STATE. 1954. *New Program for Community Mental Health Services.* Dept. of Mental Hygiene, Albany, N.Y.

102 WHO. 1959. Conference on Mental Hygiene Practice (Helsinki, 1959). Report of Committee B: Community Psychiatric Services. WHO Regional Office for Europe, Copenhagen. (Duplicated document.)

SURVEYS AND EPIDEMIOLOGICAL STUDIES

103 BLACKER, C. P. 1946. *Neurosis and the Mental Health Services.* London.

104 FELIX, R. H. & KRAMER, M. 1953. 'Extent of the problem of mental disorders.' *Ann. Amer. Acad. polit. soc. Sci.* 1953: 5–14.

105 FREMMING, K. H. 1947. *Morbid Risk of Mental Diseases in an Average Danish Population.* Copenhagen. (Also published as: *The Expectation of Mental Infirmity in a Sample of a Danish Population.* London, 1951.)

106 HALLGREN,B.&SJÖGREN,T. 1959. 'A clinical and genetico-statistical study of schizophrenia and low-grade mental deficiency in a large Swedish rural population.' *Acta psychiat.* **35**, *Suppl.* 140. Copenhagen.

107 HOCH,P.H.&ZUBIN,J. (eds.) 1961. *Comparative Epidemiology of the Mental Disorders* (Proc. 49th Ann. Meeting Amer. Psychopathol. Ass., 1959). New York.

108 HUGHES, C. C. et al. 1960. *People of Cove and Woodlot* (*The Stirling County Study of Psychiatric Disorder and Socio-cultural Environment,* Vol. 2). New York.

109 JACO, E. G. 1960. *The Social Epidemiology of Mental Disorders: A Psychiatric Survey of Texas.* New York.

110 KRAMER, M. 1953. 'Long-range studies of mental hospital patients, an important area for research in chronic disease.' *Milbank mem. Fund Quart.* **31**: 253–64.

111 KRAMER, M.1957. 'A discussion of the concepts of incidence and prevalence as related to epidemiologic studies of mental disorders.' *Amer. J. publ. Hlth* 47: 826–40.

112 LEIGHTON, A. H. 1959. *My Name is Legion (The Stirling County Study of Psychiatric Disorder and Sociocultural Environment*, Vol. 1). New York.

113 MURPHY, J. M. 1962. 'Cross-cultural studies of the prevalence of psychiatric disorders.' *World ment. Hlth* 14: 53–65.

114 NORRIS, V. 1959. *Mental Illness in London* (Maudsley Monogr. No. 6). London.

115 OPLER, M. K. 1958. 'Epidemiological studies of mental illness: methods and scope of the Midtown study in New York' In *Symposium on Preventive and Social Psychiatry* (April 1957). Walter Reed Army Institute of Research, Washington, D.C. Pp. 111–47.

116 PASAMANICk, B. (ed.) 1959. *Epidemiology of Mental Disorder*. Amer. Ass. Advanc. Sci., Washington, D.C.

117 PASAMANICK, B. 1961. 'Survey of mental disease in urban population: IV. Approach to total prevalence rates.' *Arch. gen. Psychiatr.* 5: 151–5.

118 PLUNKETT, R. J. & GORDON, J. E. 1960. *Epidemiology and Mental Illness*. New York.

119 PRIMROSE, E. J. R. 1962. *Psychological Illness: A Community Study*. (Re: General practice.) London.

120 REID, D. D. 1960. *Epidemiological Methods in the Study of Mental Disorders* (World Hlth Org. publ. Hlth Papers 2). Geneva.

121 RÜMKE, H. C. 1961. 'Identification of mental disorder and its causes.' In *Planning and Action for Mental Health*, ed. E. M. Thornton. WFMH, London. Pp. 222–8.

122 SHEPHERD, M. 1957. *A Study of the Major Psychoses in an English County* (Maudsley Monogr. No. 3). London.

123 SJÖGREN, T. & LARSSON, T. 1959. 'The changing age-structure in Sweden and its impact on mental illness.' *Bull. World Hlth. Org.* 21: 569–82.

124 SROLE, L. *et al.* 1962. *Mental Health in the Metropolis* (Midtown Manhattan Study). New York.

125 ZUBIN, J. (ed.) 1961. *Field Studies in the Mental Disorders* (Proc. Work Conf., Amer. Psychopathol. Ass., 1959). New York.

126 GROUP FOR THE ADVANCEMENT OF PSYCHIATRY (GAP). 1961. *Problems of Estimating Changes in Frequency in Mental Disorders.* Report No. 50. New York.

127 JAPAN. 1959. Report of the statistical survey of the mentally disordered in 1954. Ministry of Health & Welfare, Tokyo. (Duplicated document.)

128 MILBANK MEMORIAL FUND. 1950. *Epidemiology of Mental Disorder.* New York.

129 WHO. 1960. Epidemiology of Mental Disorders: 8th Report of the Expert Committee on Mental Health. *World Hlth Org. tech. Rep. Ser.* 185. Geneva.

130 WHO. 1961. 'The epidemiology of mental disorders.' *World Hlth Org. Chron.* **15**: 68.

CLINICAL ACTION IN THE COMMUNITY

131 AHRENFELDT, R. H. 1958. *Psychiatry in the British Army in the Second World War.* London & New York.

132 ibid. 'Practical Considerations on the Disposal of Delinquents in the Army.' Appendix A, pp. 264–8.

133 BIERER, J. 1960. 'Past, present and future.' *Int. J. soc. Psychiat.* **6**: 165–73.

134 BIERER, J. 1961. 'Day hospitals: further developments.' *Int. J. soc. Psychiat.* **7**: 148–51.

135 EHRHARDT, H. *et al.* (eds.) 1958. *Psychiatrie und Gesellschaft: Ergebnisse und Probleme der Sozialpsychiatrie.* Bern & Stuttgart.

136 FERGUSON, R. S. 1961. 'Side-effects of community care.' *Lancet* **1**: 931–2.

137 GINZBERG, E. *et al.* 1959. *The Ineffective Soldier: Lessons for Management and the Nation.* Vol. 1: *The Lost Divisions;*

Vol. 2: *Breakdown and Recovery*; Vol. 3: *Patterns of Performance*. 3 vols. New York.

138 GREENBLATT, M., LEVINSON, D. J. & KLERMAN, G. J. 1961. *Mental Patients in Transition*. Springfield, Ill.

139 HORDER, J. 1961. The Role of Public Health Officers and General Practitioners in Mental Health Care (Working Paper No. 1, May 1961). WHO Expert Committee on Mental Health, Geneva, Oct.–Nov. 1961. (Duplicated document.)

140 JONES, M. 1961. 'Intra and extramural community psychiatry.' *Amer. J. Psychiat.* 117: 748–7.

141 JONES, M. & RAPOPORT, R. N. 1955. 'Administrative and social psychiatry.' *Lancet* 2: 386–8.

142 LEIGHTON, A. H., CLAUSEN, J. A. & WILSON, R. N. (eds.) 1957. *Explorations in Social Psychiatry*. New York.

143 MACMILLAN, D. 1958. 'Community treatment of mental illness.' *Lancet* 2: 201–4.

144 MACMILLAN, D. 1961. 'Community mental health services and the mental hospital.' *World ment. Hlth* 13: 46–58.

145 MAY, A. R. 1961. 'Prescribing community care for the mentally ill.' *Lancet* 1: 760–1.

146 MCKERRACHER, D. G. 1961. 'Psychiatric care in transition.' *Ment. Hyg.* 45: 3–9.

147 REES, T. P. 1957. 'Back to moral treatment and community care.' *J. ment. Sci.* 103: 303–13.

148 ROLLIN, H. R. 1960. 'Social psychiatry in Britain.' *Trans. Coll. Physicians Philad. Ser. 4*, 27: 126–37.

149 TITMUSS, R. M. 1961. As reported in *Lancet* 1: 609.

150 VEIL, C. 1959. 'Introduction à la psychiatrie sociale.' *Bull. Centre Etudes Rech. psychotech.* 8: 29–38.

151 'Doubtful progress in psychiatry' (Correspondence). 1960. *Lancet* 2: 261, 371, 433, 599–600.

152 ENGLAND & WALES. 1951. *Report of the Committee on Social Workers in the Mental Health Services*. Ministry of Health, London.

153 WHO. 1954. *European Seminar on Mental Health Aspects of*

Public Health Practice (Amsterdam, 1953). WHO Regional Office for Europe, Geneva.

154 WHO. 1955. 'Mental health through public health practice.' *World Hlth Org. Chron.* **9**: 247–53.

155 WHO. 1959. Social Psychiatry and Community Attitudes: 7th Report of the Expert Committee on Mental Health. *World Hlth Org. tech. Rep. Ser.* 177. Geneva.

THE PSYCHIATRIC HOSPITAL

I. *Changing Patterns of Organization*

156 BAKER, A. A. 1958. 'Breaking up the mental hospital.' *Lancet* **2**: 253–5.

157 BAKER, A. A., DAVIES, R. L. & SIVADON, P. 1959. *Psychiatric Services and Architecture.* (World Hlth Org. publ. Hlth Papers 1). Geneva.

158 BARR, A., GOLDING, D. & PARNELL, R. W. 1962. 'Recent critical trends in mental hospital admissions in the Oxford Region.' *J. ment Sci.* **108**: 59–67.

159 BARTON, R., ELKES, A. & GLEN, F. 1961. 'Unrestricted visiting in a mental hospital: An inquiry into its effects and nursing-staff attitudes.' *Lancet* **1**: 1220–2.

160 BATEMAN, J. F. 1949. In *Better Care in Mental Hospitals* (Proc. 1st Mental Hospital Institute, Amer. Psychiat. Ass.). Washington, D.C. Appendix III, p. 187.

161 BERESFORD, C. 1959. Annual Report of The Retreat mental hospital, York, for 1959 – as quoted in *Lancet* **2**: 680.

162 BRIDGMAN, R. F. 1955. *The Rural Hospital: Its Structure and Organization* (World Hlth Org. Monogr. Ser. 21). Geneva.

163 CLARK, D. H. 1958. 'Administrative therapy: Its clinical importance in the mental hospital.' *Lancet* **1**: 805–8.

164 COOPER, A. B. & EARLY, D. F. 1961. 'Evolution in the mental hospital: Review of a hospital population.' *Brit. med. J.* **1**: 1600–3.

165 FLECK, S. *et al.* 1957. 'Interaction between hospital staff and families.' *Psychiatry* **20**: 343–50.

166 GARRATT, F. N., LOWE, C. R. & MCKEOWN, T. 1958. 'Institutional care of the mentally ill.' *Lancet* 1: 682–4.

167 GREENBLATT, M. *et al.* 1955. *From Custodial to Therapeutic Patient Care in Mental Hospitals.* New York. (Cf. 'Relation of the hospital to the community.' Pp. 212–34.)

168 HARPER, J. 1959. 'Out-patient adult psychiatric clinics.' *Brit. med. J.* 1: 357–60.

169 JONES, K. & SIDEBOTHAM, R. 1962. *Mental Hospitals at Work.* London.

170 KINGSTON, F. E. 1962. 'Trends in mental-hospital population and their effect on planning.' *Lancet* 2: 49.

171 LINDSAY, J. S. B. 1962. 'Trends in mental-hospital population and their effect on planning.' *Lancet* 1: 1354–5.

172 MACMILLAN, D. 1958. 'Hospital-community relationships.' In *An Approach to the Prevention of Disability from Chronic Psychoses: The Open Mental Hospital within the Community.* Milbank Memorial Fund, New York. Pp. 29–50.

173 MAIN, T. F. 1958. 'Mothers with children in a psychiatric hospital.' *Lancet* 2: 845–7.

174 NORTON, A. 1961. 'Mental hospital ins and outs: A survey of patients admitted to a mental hospital in the past 30 years.' *Brit. med. J.* 1: 528–36.

175 OVERHOLSER, W. 1955. 'The present status of the problems of release of patients from mental hospitals.' *Psychiat. Quart.* 29: 372–80.

176 REPOND, A. 1960. 'Santé mentale et hôpital psychiatrique.' *Rev. Méd. prév.* 5: 276–98.

177 RICHTER, D. (ed.) 1950. *Perspectives in Neuropsychiatry.* London.

178 SANDS, S. L. 1959. 'Discharges from mental hospitals.' *Amer. J. Psychiat.* 115: 748–50.

179 SHAW, D. & SAMUEL, A. 1959. 'Medical administration in psychiatric hospitals.' *Lancet* 2: 170–2.

180 SIVADON, P. 1959. 'Transformation d'un service d'aliénés

de type classique en un centre de traitement actif et de ré-adaptation sociale.' *Bull. World Hlth Org.* **21**: 593–600.

181 SMITH, S. *et al.* 1960. 'Metamorphosis of a mental hospital.' *Lancet* **2**: 592–3.

182 TOOTH, G. C. 1958. 'The psychiatric hospital and its place in a mental health service.' *Bull. World Hlth Org.* **19**: 363–87.

183 TOOTH, G. C. & BROOKE, E.M. 1961. 'Trends in the mental hospital population and their effect on future planning.' *Lancet* **1**: 710–13.

184 'A different hospital.' 1959. *Lancet* **2**: 221–2.

185 'A look at mental hospitals.' 1962. *Lancet* **1**: 900.

186 ENGLAND & WALES. 1962. *A Hospital Plan for England and Wales.* London.
(Preface and general review reprinted verbatim in *Brit. med. J.* 1962, **1**: 244–51.)

187 'Gains in outpatient psychiatric services, 1959.' 1960. *Publ. Hlth Rep.* **75**: 1092–4. Washington, D.C.

188 'Hospital services for the mentally ill.' 1961. *Brit. med. J.* **1**: 1184.

II. *The Therapeutic Community*

189 CAUDILL, W. 1958. *The Psychiatric Hospital as a Small Society.* Cambridge, Mass.

190 CROCKET, R. W. 1960. 'Doctors, administrators, and therapeutic communities.' *Lancet* **2**: 359–63.

191 JONES, M. *et al.* 1952. *Social Psychiatry: A Study of Therapeutic Communities.* London.

192 MAIN, T. F. 1946. 'The hospital as a therapeutic institution.' *Bull. Menninger Clin.* **10**: 66–70.

193 STANTON, A. H. & SCHWARTZ, M. S. 1954. *The Mental Hospital: A Study of Institutional Participation in Psychiatric Illness and Treatment.* New York.

194 WALTER REED ARMY INSTITUTE OF RESEARCH. 1958. 'Panel on the development of a therapeutic milieu in the mental hospital.' In *Symposium on Preventive and Social Psychiatry (April 1957).* Washington, D.C. Pp. 455–529.

195 WHO. 1953. Expert Committee on Mental Health: 3rd Report. *World Hlth Org. tech. Rep. Ser. 73.* Geneva.

III. *Day and Night Hospitals*
196 BIERER, J. 1951. *The Day Hospital: An Experiment in Social Psychiatry and Syntho-Analytic Psychotherapy.* London.
197 BIERER, J. 1959. 'Theory and practice of psychiatric day hospitals.' *Lancet* 2: 901-2.
198 BIERER, J. & BROWNE, I. W. 1960. 'An experiment with a psychiatric night hospital.' *Proc. R. Soc. Med.* 53: 930-2.
199 BOAG, T. J. 1960. 'Further developments in the day hospital.' *Amer. J. Psychiat.* 116: 801-6.
200 CAMERON, D. E. 1956. 'The day hospital.' In *The Practice of Psychiatry in General Hospitals* by A. E. Bennett et al. Berkeley & Los Angeles, Calif. Pp. 134-50.
201 CRAFT, M. 1959. 'Psychiatric day hospitals.' *Amer. J. Psychiat.* 116: 251-4.
202 FARNDALE, J. 1961. *The Day Hospital Movement in Great Britain.* Oxford.
203 FOX, R. et al. 1960. 'Psychiatric day hospitals.' *Lancet* 1: 824-5.
204 FREEMAN, H. L. 1960. 'The day hospital.' *World ment. Hlth* 12: 192-8.
205 GOSHEN, G. E. 1959. 'New concepts of psychiatric care with special reference to the day hospital.' *Amer. J. Psychiat.* 115: 808-11.

IV. *Rehabilitation*
206 BRIDGER, H. 1946. 'The Northfield experiment.' *Bull. Menninger Clin.* 10: 71-6.
207 GRAYSON, M. et al. 1952. *Psychiatric Aspects of Rehabilitation.* New York Univ., Bellevue Med. Center, New York.
208 GREENBLATT, M. & SIMON, B. (eds.) 1959. *Rehabilitation of the Mentally Ill.* Amer. Ass. Advanc. Sci., Washington, D.C.

209 LE GUILLANT, L. *et al.* 1958. 'Une réforme de l'assistance psychiatrique: Le service médico-social de secteur.' *Tech. hosp.* **14**: 34.

210 WHO. 1958. Expert Committee on Medical Rehabilitation: 1st Report. *World Hlth Org. tech. Rep. Ser.* 158. Geneva.

PSYCHOTHERAPY

211 FERENCZI, S. 1955. *Final Contributions to the Problems and Methods of Psycho-Analysis* (ed. M. Balint). London. P. 141.

212 FROMM-REICHMANN, F. & MORENO, J. L. (eds.) (Vol. 1); MASSERMAN, J. H. & MORENO, J. L. (eds.) (Vols. 2–5). 1956–60. *Progress in Psychotherapy.* 5 vols. New York.

213 MASSERMAN, J. H. & MORENO, J. L. (eds.) 1959. *Progress in Psychotherapy*, Vol 4: *Social Psychotherapy*. New York.

PHARMACOTHERAPY

214 BRILL, H. & PATTON, R. E. 1959. 'Analysis of population reduction in New York State mental hospitals during the first four years of large scale therapy with psychotropic drugs.' *Amer. J. Psychiat.* **116**: 495–509.

215 GARATTINI, S. & GHETTI, V. (eds.) 1957. *Psychotropic Drugs* (Proc. Int. Symposium on Psychotropic Drugs, Milan 1957). Amsterdam.

216 GELBER, I. 1959. *Release Mental Patients on Tranquillizing Drugs and the Public Health Nurse.* New York.

217 GROSS, M. 1960. 'The impact of ataractic drugs on a mental hospital out-patient clinic.' *Amer. J. Psychiat.* **117**, 444–7.

218 GUPTA, J. C., DEB, A. K. & KAHALI, B. S. 1943. 'Preliminary observations on the use of *Rauwolfia serpentina* Benth. in the treatment of mental disorders.' *Indian med. Gaz.* **78**: 547–9.

219 HOCH, P. H. 1959. 'Drug therapy.' In *American Handbook of Psychiatry*, ed. S. Arieti. New York. Vol. 2: 1541–51.

220 HUTCHINSON, J. T. & SMEDBERG, D. 1960. 'Phenelzine ("Nardil") in the treatment of endogenous depression.' *J. ment. Sci.* **106**: 704–10.

221 HUTCHINSON, R. 1953. 'Modern treatment.' *Brit. med J.* **1**: 671.

222 JACOBSEN, E. 1959. 'The comparative pharmacology of some psychotropic drugs.' *Bull. World Hlth Org.* **21**: 411–93.

223 KILOH, L. G. & BALL, J. R. B. 1961. 'Depression treated with imipramine ("Tofranil"): A follow-up study.' *Brit. med. J.* **1**: 168–71.

224 KLINE, N. S. 1959. 'Psychopharmaceuticals: Effects and side-effects.' *Bull. World Hlth Org.* **21**: 397–410.

225 KLINE, N. S. (ed.) 1959. *Psychopharmacology Frontiers* (2nd Int. Congr. Psychiatry: Proc. Psychopharmacol. Symposium). Boston.

226 LINDEMANN, E. 1959. 'The relation of drug-induced mental changes to psychoanalytical theory.' *Bull. World Hlth Org.* **21**: 517–26.

227 LINN, E. L. 1959. 'Sources of uncertainty in studies of drugs affecting mood, mentation or activity.' *Amer. J. Psychiat.* **116**: 97–103.

228 PRINCE, R. 1960. 'The use of *Rauwolfia* for the treatment of psychoses by Nigerian native doctors.' *Amer. J. Psychiat.* **117**: 147–9.

229 REES, L., BROWN, A. C. & BENAIM, S. 1961. 'A controlled trial of imipramine ("Tofranil") in the treatment of severe depressive states.' *J. ment. Sci.* **107**: 552–9.

230 REES, L. & DAVIES, B. 1961. 'A controlled trial of phenelzine ("Nardil") in the treatment of severe depressive illness.' *J. ment. Sci.* **107**: 560–6.

231 SANDISON, R. A. 1959. 'The role of psychotropic drugs in group therapy.' *Bull. World Hlth Org.* **21**: 505–15.

232 SANDISON, R. A. 1959. 'The role of psychotropic drugs in individual therapy.' *Bull. World Hlth Org.* **21**: 495–503.

233 UHR, L. & MILLER, J. G. (eds.) 1960. *Drugs and Behavior.* New York.

234 WATT, J. M. & BREYER-BRANDWIJK, M. G. 1962. *The Medicinal and Poisonous Plants of Southern and Eastern Africa*. (2nd ed.) Edinburgh. Pp. 95–100.

235 PIUS XII. 1960. 'Psychiatrie et psychopharmacologie (1958).' In *Pie XII parle de santé mentale et de psychologie*. Bruxelles. Pp. 72–75 (and cf. E. E. Krapf, Préface, p. 10).

236 WHO. 1958. Ataractic and Hallucinogenic Drugs in Psychiatry; Report of a Study Group. *World Hlth Org. tech. Rep. Ser.* 152. Geneva.

PSYCHIATRY IN THE GENERAL HOSPITAL

237 BENNETT, E. A. *et al.* 1956. *The Practice of Psychiatry in General Hospitals*. Berkeley & Los Angeles, Calif.

238 BENNETT, A. E. 1959. 'Problems in establishing and maintaining psychiatric units in general hospitals.' *Amer. J. Psychiat.* 115: 974–9.

239 BROOK, C. P. B. & STAFFORD-CLARK, D. 1961. 'Psychiatric treatment in general wards.' *Lancet* 1: 1159–62.

240 COHEN, N. A. & HALDANE, F. P. 1962. 'Inpatient psychiatry in general hospitals.' *Lancet* 1: 1113–14.

241 COTTON, J. M. 1961. 'The function of a psychiatric service in a general hospital.' *Mental Hosp.*, Sept., pp. 4–7.

242 HOENIG, J. & CROTTY, I. M. 1959. 'Psychiatric inpatients in general hospitals.' *Lancet* 2: 122–3.

243 LINN, L. 1955. *A Handbook of Hospital Psychiatry: A Practical Guide to Therapy*. New York.

244 LINN, L. (ed.) 1961. *Frontiers in General Hospital Psychiatry*. New York.

245 MOROSS, H. 1954. 'The administration of a psychiatric service in a general hospital.' *S. Afr. med. J.* 28: 886–9.

246 NOBLE, H. N. 1961. As reported in *Brit. med. J.* 1: 664–5.

247 SMITH, S. 1961. 'Psychiatry in general hospitals: Manchester's integrated scheme.' *Lancet* 1: 1158–9.

248 'Psychiatry in the general hospital.' 1962. *Lancet* 1: 1107.

PSYCHIATRY IN OBSTETRIC PRACTICE

249 HARGREAVES, G. R. 1955. 'Obstetrics and psychiatry.' *Lancet* 1: 39-40.

250 MORRIS, N. 1960. 'Human relations in obstetric practice.' *Lancet* 1: 913-15.

251 ENGLAND & WALES. 1961. *Human Relations in Obstetrics.* Ministry of Health, London.

PSYCHIATRY IN GENERAL PRACTICE

252 BALINT, M. 1957. *The Doctor, his Patient and the Illness.* London.

253 FRANKLIN, L. M. 1960. 'An appraisal of psychiatry in general practice.' *Brit. med. J.* 2: 451-3.

254 KRAPF, E. E. 1956. 'Tâches et possibilités du médecin de famille dans le domaine de l'hygiène mentale.' *Arch. suisses Neurol. Psychiat.* 77: 47-56.
(English transl.: 'The family doctor's tasks and opportunities in the field of mental hygiene.' *J. Amer. med. Women's Ass.*, 1957, 12: 212-15.)

255 LEMERE, F. & KRAABEL, A. B. 1959. 'The general practitioner and the psychiatrist.' *Amer. J. Psychiat.* 116: 518-521.

256 WATTS, C. A. H. 1958. 'Management of chronic psychoneurosis in general practice.' *Lancet* 2: 362-4.

257 COLLEGE OF GENERAL PRACTITIONERS. 1958. 'Psychological medicine in general practice.' *Brit. med. J.* 2: 585-90.

THE MENTAL HEALTH OF THE GENERAL HOSPITAL

258 BARNES, E. 1959. 'Mental health in general hospitals.' *World ment. Hlth* 11: 43-7.

259 BARNES, E. 1961. *People in Hospital.* London.

260 BLUESTONE, E. M. 1958. 'Fear in hospital practice: Some advantages of home care.' *Lancet* 1: 1083-4.

261 HEASMAN, G. A. 1962. 'The patient, the doctor and the hospital.' *Lancet* 2: 59-62.

262 STATHAM, C. 1959. 'Noise and the patient in hospital: A personal investigation.' *Brit. med. J.* **2**: 1247–8.

263 ENGLAND & WALES. 1953. *The Reception and Welfare of In-Patients in Hospitals.* Ministry of Health, London.

264 ENGLAND & WALES. 1961. *The Pattern of the In-Patient's Day.* Ministry of Health, London.

265 KING EDWARD'S HOSPITAL FUND FOR LONDON. 1958. *Noise Control in Hospitals.* London.
(Cf. *Lancet*, 1958, **2**: 1269.)

266 KING EDWARD'S HOSPITAL FUND FOR LONDON. 1962. *Information Booklets for Patients.* London.
(Cf. *Lancet*, 1962, **1**: 1392–3.)

267 SCOTTISH ASS. MENTAL HEALTH. 1960. *Report of Scottish Study Group on Psychological Problems in General Hospitals.* Edinburgh.

THE MENTAL HEALTH OF CHILDREN

I. *Clinical Problems*

268 BRADLEY, C. 1941. *Schizophrenia in Childhood.* New York. Pp. 21–4.

269 BROCK, J. F. & AUTRET, M. 1952. *Kwashiorkor in Africa* (World Hlth Org. Monogr. Ser. 8). Geneva.

270 FREEDMAN, A. M. 1959. 'Day hospitals for severely schizophrenic children.' *Amer. J. Psychiat.* **115**: 893–8.

271 GEBER, M. & DEAN, R. F. A. 1955. 'Psychological factors in the aetiology of kwashiorkor.' *Bull. World Hlth Org.* **12**: 471–5.

272 JELLIFFE, D. B. 1955. *Infant Nutrition in the Subtropics and Tropics* (World Hlth Org. Monogr. Ser. 29). Geneva.

273 KANNER, L. 1959. 'Trends in child psychiatry.' *J. ment. Sci.* **105**: 581–93.

274 LORAND, S. & SCHNEER, H. I. (eds.) 1961. *Adolescents: Psychoanalytic Approach to Problems and Therapy.* New York.

275 LURIA, A. K. 1961. *The Role of Speech in the Regulation of Normal and Abnormal Behaviour* (ed. J. Tizard). Oxford.

276 MOSSE, H. L. 1958. 'The misuse of the diagnosis, childhood schizophrenia.' *Amer. J. Psychiat.* **114**: 791–4.

277 SHAGASS, C. & PASAMANICK, B. (eds.) 1960. *Child Development and Child Psychiatry.* In Tribute to Dr Arnold Gesell in his Eightieth Year. Washington, D.C.

278 SODDY, K. 1960. *Clinical Child Psychiatry.* London.

279 TANNER, J. M. & INHELDER, B. (eds.) 1956–60. *Discussions on Child Development.* 4 vols. London.

280 TIZARD, J. P. M. *et al.* 1959. 'The role of the paediatrician in mental illness.' *Lancet* **2**: 193–5.

281 AMERICAN PSYCHIATRIC ASSOCIATION. 1957. *Psychiatric Inpatient Treatment of Children.* Washington, D.C.

282 CENTRE INTERNATIONAL DE L'ENFANCE. 1953. *Les Problèmes de l'enfance dans les pays tropicaux de l'Afrique* (Brazzaville, 1952). Paris. Pp. 315–61.

II. *Organization of Services*

283 BUCKLE, D. & LEBOVICI, S. 1960. *Child Guidance Centres* (World Hlth Org. Monogr. Ser. 40). Geneva.

284 CONNELL, P. H. 1961. 'The day hospital approach in child psychiatry.' *J. ment. Sci.* **107**: 969–77.

285 CREAK, M. 1959. 'Child health and child psychiatry: neighbours or colleagues?' *Lancet* **1**: 481–5.

286 POLLAK, O. *et al.* 1952. *Social Science and Psychotherapy for Children.* New York.

287 SMALLPEICE, V. 1958. 'Children as day patients.' *Lancet* **2**: 1366–7.

288 ENGLAND & WALES. 1955. *Report of the Committee on Maladjusted Children.* Ministry of Education, London.

289 WHO. 1952. *Scandinavian Seminar on Child Psychiatry and Child Guidance Work* (Lillehammer, 1952). WHO Regional Office for Europe, Geneva.

290 WHO. 1952. Joint Expert Committee on the Physically Handicapped Child: 1st Report. *World Hlth Org. tech. Rep. Ser.* 58. Geneva.

III. *Children in Hospital*

291 CAPES, M. 1955. 'The child in hospital.' *Bull. World Hlth Org.* **12**: 427–70.

292 ILLINGWORTH, R. S. 1958. 'Children in hospital.' *Lancet* **2**: 165–71.

293 TREADGOLD, S. 1960. 'Billy goes to hospital.' *Med. biol. Illustr.* **10**: 191–6.

294 BRITISH PAEDIATRIC ASS. 1959. 'The welfare of children in hospital.' *Brit. med. J.* **1**: 166–9.

295 ENGLAND & WALES. 1959. *The Welfare of Children in Hospital.* Ministry of Health, London.

SOME SPECIFIC AREAS OF MENTAL HEALTH CONCERN

I. *Addiction*

296 DUHL, L. J. 1959. 'Alcoholism: The public health approach – A new look from the viewpoint of human ecology.' *Quart. J. Stud. Alc.* **20**: 112–25.

297 JELLINEK, E. M. 1960. *The Disease Concept of Alcoholism.* New Haven.

298 JELLINEK, E. M. *et al.* 1955. 'The "craving" for alcohol: A symposium by members of the WHO Expert Committees on Mental Health and on Alcohol.' *Quart J. Stud. Alc.* **16**: 34–66.

299 KILOH, L. G. & BRANDON, S. 1962. 'Habituation and addiction to amphetamines.' *Brit. med. J.* **2**: 40–3.

300 KRUSE, H. D. (ed.) 1961. *Alcoholism as a Medical Problem.* New York.

301 CALIFORNIA. 1961. *Reports of the Division of Alcoholic Rehabilitation of the Department of Public Health (State of California).* Publ. No. 1: A Study of Community Concepts and Definitions (Pt. I); Publ. No. 2: Selected Aspects of the Prospective Follow-up Study (a preliminary review); Publ. No. 3: Criminal Offenders and Drinking Involvement (a preliminary analysis).

302 WHO. 1951. *European Seminar and Lecture Course on Alcoholism* (Copenhagen, 1951). WHO Regional Office for Europe, Geneva.

303 WHO. 1951–55. Expert Committee on Mental Health – Alcoholism Sub-committee: 1st and 2nd Reports; Expert Committee on Alcohol: 1st Report; Alcohol and Alcoholism: Report of an Expert Committee. *World Hlth Org. tech. Rep. Ser.* 42, 48, 84, 94. Geneva.

304 WHO. 1955. *European Seminar on the Prevention and Treatment of Alcoholism*: Selected Lectures (Noordwijk, 1954). WHO Regional Office for Europe, Geneva. (Reprinted from *Quart. J. Stud. Alc.* 1954, **15**, and 1955, **16**.)

305 WHO. 1957–61. Treatment and Care of Drug Addicts: Report of a Study Group; Expert Committee on Addiction-Producing Drugs: 10th and 11th Reports. *World Hlth Org. tech. Rep. Ser.* 131, 188, 211. Geneva.

II. *Ageing*

306 ANDERSON, J. E. (ed.) 1956. *Psychological Aspects of Aging.* Amer. Psychol. Ass., Washington, D.C.

307 BASH, K. W. 1959. 'Mental health problems of aging and the aged from the viewpoint of analytical psychology.' *Bull. World Hlth Org.* **21**: 563–8.

308 COSIN, L. Z. 1955. 'The place of the day hospital in the geriatric unit.' *Int. J. soc. Psychiat.* **1**: No. 2, 33–41.

309 HARGREAVES, G. R. *et al.* 1962. 'Psychiatric and geriatric beds' (Central Consultants and Specialists Committee). As reported in *Brit. med. J., Suppl.* **1**: 209–10.

310 HOCH, P. H. & ZUBIN, J. (eds.) 1961. *Psychopathology of Aging* (Proc. 50th Ann. Meeting Amer. Psychopathol. Ass., 1960). New York.

311 ROTH, M. 1959. 'Mental health problems of aging and the aged.' *Bull. World Hlth Org.* **21**: 527–61, 563–91.

312 SHELDON, J. H. 1960. 'Problems of an ageing population. *Brit. med. J.* **1**: 1223–30.

313 WHO. 1959. Mental Health Problems of Aging and the Aged: 6th Report of the Expert Committee on Mental Health. *World Hlth Org. tech. Rep. Ser.* 171. Geneva.

III. *Cyclothymia*

314 GIBSON, R. W. *et al.* 1959. 'On the dynamics of the manic-depressive personality.' *Amer. J. Psychiat.* 115: 1101–7.

315 STENSTEDT, A. 1959. 'Involutional melancholia: An etiologic, clinical and social study of endogenous depression in later life, with special reference to genetic factors.' *Acta psychiat.* 34, *Suppl.* 127, Copenhagen.

IV. *Delinquency and Criminality*

316 BOVET, L. 1951. *Psychiatric Aspects of Juvenile Delinquency* (World Hlth Org. Monogr. Ser. 1). Geneva.

317 EDELSTON, H. 1952. *The Earliest Stages of Delinquency: A Clinical Study from the Child Guidance Clinic.* Edinburgh.

318 GIBBENS, T. C. N. 1961. *Trends in Juvenile Delinquency* (World Hlth Org. publ. Hlth Papers 5). Geneva.

319 GITTINS, J. 1952. *Approved School Boys: An Account of the Observation, Classification and Treatment of Boys who come to Aycliffe School.* Home Office, London. (Cf. esp. Pt. III, pp. 84 ff., on psychiatric and psychometric investigations.)

320 JONES, H. 1960. *Reluctant Rebels: Re-education and Group Process in a Residential Community.* London.

321 MANNHEIM, H. & WILKINS, L. T. 1955. *Prediction Methods in Relation to Borstal Training.* London.

V. *Migration*

322 EITINGER, L. 1960. 'The symptomatology of mental disease among refugees in Norway.' *J. ment. Sci.* 106: 947–66.

323 LISTWAN, I. A. 1959. 'Mental disorders in migrants: Further study.' *Med. J. Australia,* April. (Reprinted in *World ment. Hlth,* 1960, 12: 38–45.)

324 MEZEY, A. G. 1960. 'Personal background, emigration and mental disorder in Hungarian refugees.' *J. ment. Sci.* **106**: 618–27.

325 MEZEY, A. G. 1960. 'Psychiatric aspects of human migrations.' *Int. J. soc. Psychiat.* **5**: 245–60.

326 MEZEY, A. G. 1960. 'Psychiatric illness in Hungarian refugees.' *J. ment Sci.* **106**: 628–37.

VI. *Neurosis, and Physical and Psychosomatic Illness*

327 BARKER, R. G. *et al.* 1953. *Adjustment to Physical Handicap and Illness: A Survey of the Social Psychology of Physique and Disability.* Social Sci. Res. Council, New York.

328 BARTON, R. 1959. *Institutional Neurosis.* Bristol.

329 CLECKLEY, H. M. 1959. 'Psychopathic states.' In *American Handbook of Psychiatry*, ed. S. Arieti. New York. Vol. 1: 567–88.

330 COHEN OF BIRKENHEAD, LORD. 1958. 'Epilepsy as a social problem.' *Brit. med. J.* **1**: 672–5.

331 DERNER, G. F. 1953. *Aspects of the Psychology of the Tuberculous.* New York.

332 KRAPF, E. E. 1957. 'On the pathogenesis of epileptic and hysterical seizures.' *Bull. World Hlth Org.* **16**: 749–62.

333 LJUNGBERG, L. 1957. 'Hysteria: A clinical, prognostic and genetic study.' *Acta psychiat.* **32,** *Suppl.* 112. Copenhagen.

334 LOWINGER, P. 1959. 'Leprosy and psychosis.' *Amer. J. Psychiat.* **116**: 32–7.

335 MANSON-BAHR, P. E. C. 1960. 'The physical background of mental disorder in Africans.' *E. Afr. med. J.* **37**: 477–9.

336 MARS, L. 1955. *La Crise de possession: Essais de psychiatrie comparée.* Port-au-Prince, Haiti.

337 MILLER, H. 1961. 'Accident neurosis.' *Brit. med. J.* **1**: 919–25, 992–8.

338 TANNER, J. M. (ed.) 1960. *Stress and Psychiatric Disorder* (2nd. Oxford Conf. Ment. Health Res. Fund). Oxford.

339 WITTKOWER, E. D. 1955. *A Psychiatrist Looks at Tuberculosis.* (2nd ed.) London.

340 WITTKOWER, E. D. & CLEGHORN, R. A. (eds.) 1954. *Recent Developments in Psychosomatic Medicine.* London.

341 WITTKOWER, E. D. & RUSSELL, B. 1953. *Emotional Factors in Skin Disease.* New York.

342 YAP, P. M. 1960. 'The possession syndrome: A comparison of Hong Kong and French findings.' *J. ment. Sci.* 106: 114–37.

343 ENGLAND & WALES. 1956. *Report of the Sub-committee on the Medical Care of Epileptics.* Ministry of Health, London.

344 PIUS XII. 1960. 'Ressources psycho-spirituelles dans la réhabilitation des malades de la lèpre (1956).' In *Pie XII parle de santé mentale et de psychologie.* Bruxelles. Pp. 68–9.

345 WHO. 1957. Juvenile Epilepsy: Report of a Study Group *World Hlth Org. tech. Rep. Ser.* 130. Geneva.

346 WHO. 1961. 'Rehabilitation in leprosy.' *World Hlth Org. Chron.* 15: 111.

VII. *Schizophrenia*

347 BROWN, G. W. 1960. 'Length of stay and schizophrenia: A review of statistical studies.' *Acta psychiat.* 35: 414–30.

348 FLECK, S. 1960. 'Family dynamics and origin of schizophrenia.' *Psychosom. Med.* 22: 333–44.

349 LIDZ, T. & FLECK, S. 1959. 'Schizophrenia, human integration, and the role of the family.' In *Etiology of Schizophrenia,* ed. D. Jackson. New York. Pp. 323–45.

350 LIDZ, T. et al. 1957. 'The intrafamilial environment of the schizophrenic patient: I. The father.' *Psychiatry* 20: 329–42.

351 WING, J. K. 1960. 'Pilot experiment in the rehabilitation of long-hospitalized male schizophrenic patients.' *Brit. J. prev. soc. Med.* 14: 173–80.

352 WING, J. K. & BROWN, G. W. 1961. 'Social treatment of chronic schizophrenia: A constructive survey of three mental hospitals.' *J. ment. Sci.* 107: 847–61.

353 *Second International Congress for Psychiatry (Zürich).* 1957. *Congress Report.* Zürich. Vol. I (contains a number of papers on schizophrenia in various cultures).

354 WHO. 1959. Report of World Health Organization Study Group on Schizophrenia – Geneva, 9–14 September 1959. *Amer. J. Psychiat.* 115: 865–72.

VIII. *Subnormality*

355 ADAMS, M. (ed.) 1960. *The Mentally Subnormal: The Social Casework Approach.* London.

356 CLARKE, A. M. & CLARKE, A. D. B. (eds.) 1958. *Mental Deficiency: The Changing Outlook.* London.

357 CRAFT, M. 1959. 'Personality disorder and dullness.' *Lancet* I: 856–8.

358 EARL, C. J. C. 1961. *Subnormal Personalities: Their Clinical Investigation and Assessment*; with additional material by H. C. Gunzburg. London.

359 JERVIS, G. A. 1959. 'The mental deficiencies.' In *American Handbook of Psychiatry*, ed. S. Arieti. New York. Vol. 2: 1312–13.

360 LEWIS, A. J. 1960. 'The study of defect' (Adolf Meyer Research Lecture). *Amer. J. Psychiat.* 117: 289–305.

361 O'GORMAN, G. 1958. 'A hospital for the psychotic-defective child.' *Lancet* 2: 951–3.

362 SLAUGHTER, S. S. 1960. *The Mentally Retarded Child and his Parent.* New York.

363 TIZARD, J. 1953. 'The prevalence of mental subnormality.' *Bull. World Hlth Org.* 9: 423–40.

364 TIZARD, J. & GRAD, J. C. 1961. *The Mentally Handicapped and their Families: A Social Survey* (Maudsley Monogr. No. 7). London.

365 TOKUHATA, G. K. & STEHMAN, V. A. 1961. 'Sociologic implications, and epidemiology, of mental disorders in recent Japan.' *Amer. J. publ. Hlth* 51: 697–705.

366 WHO. 1954. The Mentally Subnormal Child. *World Hlth Org. tech. Rep. Ser.* 75. Geneva.

367 WHO. 1957. *European Seminar on the Mental Health of the Subnormal Child* (Oslo, 1957). WHO Regional Office for Europe, Copenhagen.

IX. *Suicide*

368 CAPSTICK, A. 1960. 'Urban and rural suicide.' *J. ment. Sci.* **106**: 1327–36.
369 SAINSBURY, P. 1955. *Suicide in London: An Ecological Study.* London.
370 STENGEL, E. 1960. 'The complexity of motivations to suicidal attempts.' *J. ment. Sci.* **106**: 1388–93.
371 VEIL, C. 1957. 'Note sur la gravité et l'urgence en psychiatrie de dispensaire.' *Ann. médico-psychol.* **2**: 124–7.
372 YAP, P. M. 1958. *Suicide in Hong Kong.* Hong Kong.

Preventive Aspects of Mental Health Action

PROMOTION OF MENTAL HEALTH
IN THE COMMUNITY

373 CAPLAN, G. 1961. *An Approach to Community Mental Health.* London.

374 FRASER, F. 1958. 'Medical practice in a changing society.' *Lancet* 1: 154-7.

375 GOTTLIEB, J. S. & HOWELL, R. W. 1957. 'The concepts of "prevention" and "creativity development" as applied to mental health.' In *Four Basic Aspects of Preventive Psychiatry*, ed. R. H. Ojemann. State Univ. Iowa, Iowa City. Pp. 9-17.

376 JONES, K. 1960. *Mental Health and Social Policy, 1845–1959.* London. (Cf. especially Chap. 11, 'Problems and Experiments, 1948–59'; pp. 153-77.)

377 KEBRIKOV, O. V. *et al.* 1954. *Reports of the Members of the Soviet Delegation at the Fifth Congress on Mental Health Defence.* Moscow.

378 KRAPF, E. E. 1955. 'Structure and functions of the Mental Health Society.' *Ment. Hyg.* **39**: 225-31.

379 KRAPF, E. E. 1958. 'The work of the World Health Organization in relation to the mental health problems in changing cultures.' In *Growing Up in a Changing World.* WFMH, London. Pp. 106-12.

380 KRUSE, H. D. (ed.) 1957. *Integrating the Approaches to Mental Disease.* (2 Conferences held under the auspices of the Committee of Public Health, N.Y. Acad. Med.) New York.

381 LEMKAU, P. V. 1952. 'Toward mental health: Areas that promise progress.' *Ment. Hyg.* **36**: 197-209.

382 MACMILLAN, D. 1960. 'Preventive geriatrics: Opportunities of a community mental health service.' *Lancet* 2: 1439-41.

383 SIVADON, P. & DUCHÊNE, H. 1958. 'Santé mentale, hygiène mentale et prophylaxie mentale.' In *Traité de psychiatrie: Encyclopédie médico-chirurgicale*. Paris. Tome 3, art. 37960 A30, p. 3.

384 STEVENSON, G. S. 1956. *Mental Health Planning for Social Action*. New York.

385 TUFTS, E. M. 1955. 'The field of mental health promotion.' In *Community Programs for Mental Health*, ed. R. Kotinsky & H. L. Witmer. Cambridge, Mass. Pp. 33–45.

386 WILLIAMS, C. D. 1958. 'Social medicine in developing countries.' *Lancet* 1: 863–6, 919–22.

387 *Constructive Mental Hygiene in the Caribbean* (Proc. 1st Caribbean Conf. on Mental Health, March 1957). Assen.

388 MILBANK MEMORIAL FUND. 1956. *The Elements of a Community Mental Health Program*. New York. Pp. 101–5 & 122–34.
(G. R. Hargreaves: The Protection of the Personality.)

389 UNITED STATES. 1961. Joint Commission on Mental Illness and Health, *Action for Mental Health*. New York. (Cf. Summary, 'Action for Mental Health: Digest of Final Report.' *Modern Hosp.*, 1961, **96**, 109–24.)

390 WHO. 1957. The Psychiatric Hospital as a Centre for Preventive Work in Mental Health: 5th Report of the Expert Committee on Mental Health. *World Hlth Org. tech. Rep. Ser.* 134. Geneva.

391 WHO. 1961. Programme Development in the Mental Health Field: 10th Report of the Expert Committee on Mental Health. *World Hlth Org. tech. Rep. Ser.* 223. Geneva.

PUBLIC HEALTH IN ACTION

392 GRUENBERG, E. M. 1957. 'Application of control methods to mental illness.' *Amer. J. publ. Hlth.* **47**: 944–52.

393 HARGREAVES, G. R. 1958. *Psychiatry and the Public Health*. London.

394 LEMKAU, P. V. 1955. *Mental Hygiene in Public Health*. (2nd ed.) New York. Pp. 11 et seq.

395 UNITED KINGDOM. 1956. *An Inquiry into Health Visiting: Report of a Working Party on the Field of Work, Training and Recruitment of Health Visitors.* Ministry of Health, Dept of Health for Scotland, and Ministry of Education, London.

LEGISLATION

396 DAVIDSON, H. A. 1959. 'The commitment procedures and their legal implications.' In *American Handbook of Psychiatry,* ed. S. Arieti. New York. Vol 2: 1902–22.

397 GOTTLIEB, J. S. & TOURNEY, G. 1958. 'Commitment procedures and the advancement of psychiatric knowledge.' *Amer. J. Psychiat.* **115**: 109–13.

398 GRAY, H. R. 1960. 'The reform of the law relating to mental health.' *New Zealand med. J.* **59**: 18–23.

399 MACLAY, W. S. 1960. 'The new Mental Health Act in England and Wales.' *Amer. J. Psychiat.* **116**: 777–81.

400 ENGLAND & WALES. 1948. *National Health Service Act, 1946: Provisions Relating to the Mental Health Services.* Ministry of Health, London.

401 SCOTLAND. 1955. *The Law Relating to Mental Illness and Mental Deficiency in Scotland: Proposals for Amendment.* Dept of Health, Edinburgh.

402 SCOTLAND. 1959. *Mental Health Legislation: 2nd Report by a Committee appointed by the Council.* Dept. of Health & Scottish Health Services Council, Edinburgh.

403 'The Mental Health Act.' 1960. *Brit. med. J.* **2**: 1297–8.

404 UNITED KINGDOM. 1957. *Royal Commission on the Law relating to Mental Illness and Mental Deficiency, 1954–1957: Report.* London.

405 WHO. 1955. *Hospitalization of Mental Patients: A Survey of Existing Legislation.* Geneva.

406 WHO. 1955. Legislation Affecting Psychiatric Treatment: 4th Report of the Expert Committee on Mental Health. *World Hlth Org. tech. Rep. Ser.* 98. Geneva.

MENTAL HEALTH IN INFANCY

407 BOWLBY, J. 1951. *Maternal Care and Mental Health* (World Hlth Org. Monogr. Ser. 2). Geneva.

408 BOWLBY, J. 1958. 'Separation of mother and child.' *Lancet* 1: 480.

409 BOWLBY, J. 1958. 'The nature of the child's tie to his mother.' *Int. J. Psycho-Anal.* **39**: 350–73.

410 FOSS, B. M. (ed.) 1961. *Determinants of Infant Behaviour: Proceedings of a Tavistock Study Group on Mother-Infant Interaction* (Ciba Foundation, Sept. 1959). London.

411 MEAD, M. 1954. 'Some theoretical considerations on the problem of mother-child separation.' *Amer. J. Orthopsychiat.* **24**: 471–83.

412 MURPHY, L. B. *et al.* 1956. *Personality in Young Children.* 2 vols. New York.

413 STONE, F. H. 1958. 'Early disorders of the mother-child relationship.' *Lancet* 1: 1115–18.

414 'Problèmes d'hygiène mentale posés par la séparation des jeunes enfants de leur mère.' 1957. *Hyg. Ment.* No 1.

415 WHO. 1962. *Deprivation of Maternal Care: A Reassessment of its Effects* (World Hlth Org. publ. Hlth Papers 14). Geneva.

THE WELFARE OF CHILDREN

416 BACKETT, E. M. & JOHNSTON, A. M. 1959. 'Social patterns of road accidents to children: Some characteristics of vulnerable families.' *Brit. med. J.* 1: 409–13.

417 BAUCHARD, P. 1953. *The Child Audience: A Report on Press, Film and Radio for Children.* UNESCO, Paris.

418 CAPLAN, G. (ed.) 1961. *Prevention of Mental Disorder in Children: Initial Explorations.* London.

419 DUHRSSEN, A. 1958. *Heimkinder und Pflegekinder in ihrer Entwicklung.* Göttingen.

420 GINZBERG, E. (ed.) 1960. *The Nation's Children.* Vols 1 & 3. New York.

421 HIMMELWEIT, H. T. *et al.* 1958. *Television and the Child.* London.

422 HOCHFELD, E. & VALK, M. A. 1953. *Experience in Inter-Country Adoptions.* Int. Social Service (Amer. Branch), New York.

423 WERTHAM, F. 1954. *Seduction of the Innocent.* New York.

424 ENGLAND & WALES. 1955. *Seventh Report on the Work of the Children's Department: November 1955.* Home Office, London.

425 ENGLAND & WALES. 1960. *Report of the Committee on Children and Young Persons.* Home Office, London.

426 UNITED KINGDOM. 1954. *Report of the Departmental Committee on the Adoption of Children.* Home Office & Scottish Home Dept, London.

427 WHO. 1953. Joint UN/WHO Meeting of Experts on the Mental Health Aspects of Adoption: Final Report. *World Hlth Org. tech. Rep. Ser.* 70. Geneva.

428 WHO. 1957. Accidents in Childhood: Facts as a Basis for Prevention – Report of an Advisory Group. *World Hlth Org. tech. Rep. Ser.* 118. Geneva.

429 WHO. 1959. 'Accidents in childhood in the Americas.' *World Hlth Org. Chron.* 13: 249–50.

430 WHO. 1960. *Seminar on the Prevention of Accidents in Childhood* (Spa, 1958). WHO Regional Office for Europe, Copenhagen.

THE FAMILY

431 ACKERMAN, N. W. *The Psychodynamics of Family Life.* New York.

432 BLACKER, C. P. 1958. 'Disruption of marriage: Some possibilities of prevention.' *Lancet* 1: 578–81.

433 EISENSTEIN, V. W. (ed.) 1956. *Neurotic Interaction in Marriage.* New York.

434 LIN, T. (ed.) 1960. *Reality and Vision: A Report of the First Asian Seminar on Mental Health and Family Life* (Baguio, 1958). Manila.

MENTAL HEALTH AND THE EDUCATIONAL SYSTEM

435 ANDERSON, H. H. *et al.* 1959. 'Image of the teacher by adolescent children in four countries: Germany, England, Mexico, United States.' *J. soc. Psychol.* **50**: 47–55.

436 BONNEY, M. E. 1960. *Mental Health in Education.* Boston.

437 BOWER, E. M. 1960. *Early Identification of Emotionally Handicapped Children in School.* Springfield, Ill.

438 KAPLAN, L. 1959. *Mental Health and Human Relations in Education.* New York.

439 KRUGMAN, M. (ed.) 1958. *Orthopsychiatry and the School.* New York.

440 MACFARLANE, J. W. 1953. 'The uses and predictive limitations of intelligence tests in infants and young children.' *Bull. World Hlth Org.* **9**: 409–15.

441 SHIPLEY, J. T. 1961. *The Mentally Disturbed Teacher.* Philadelphia.

442 WALL, W. D. 1955. *Education and Mental Health* (Problems in Education XI). UNESCO, Paris.

443 WHEELER, O., PHILLIPS, W. & SPILLANE, J. P. 1961. *Mental Health and Education.* London.

444 ENGLAND & WALES. 1952. *The Health of the School Child: Report of the Chief Medical Officer of the Ministry of Education for 1950 and 1951.* Ministry of Education, London.

445 SCOTTISH COUNCIL FOR RESEARCH IN EDUCATION. 1953. *Social Implications of the 1947 Scottish Mental Survey.*

446 SCOTTISH COUNCIL FOR RESEARCH IN EDUCATION. 1959. *Educational . . . Aspects of the 1947 Scottish Mental Survey.*

447 WHO. 1951. Expert Committee on School Health Services: Report on the 1st Session. *World Hlth Org. tech. Rep. Ser.* **30**: pp. 14–16. Geneva.

STUDENT MENTAL HEALTH

448 BLAINE, G. & MACARTHUR, C. 1961. *Emotional Problems of the Student.* New York.

449 DAVIDSON, M. A. *et al.* 1955. 'The detection of psychological vulnerability in students.' *J. ment. Sci.* **101**: 810–25.

450 DAVY, B. W. 1960. 'The sources and prevention of mental ill-health in university students.' *Proc. R. Soc. Med.* **53**: 764–9.

451 FARNSWORTH, D. L. 1957. *Mental Health in College and University.* Cambridge, Mass.

452 FARNSWORTH, D. L. 1959. 'Social and emotional development of students in college and university.' *Ment. Hyg.* **43**: 358–67, 568–76.

453 FUNKENSTEIN, D. H. (ed.) 1959. *The Student and Mental Health: An International View* (Proc. 1st Int. Conf. Student Mental Health, Princeton, 1956). Cambridge, Mass.

454 FUNKENSTEIN, D. H. & WILKIE, G. H. 1956. *Student Mental Health: An annotated Bibliography, 1936–1955.* WFMH, London; Int. Ass. Universities, Paris.

455 PRINCE, R. 1960. 'The "brain fag" syndrome in Nigerian students.' *J. ment. Sci.* **106**: 559–70.

456 ROOK, A. 1959. 'Student suicides.' *Brit. med. J.* **1**: 599–603.

457 WAGGONER, R. W. & ZEIGLER, T. W. 1961. 'Psychiatric factors in medical students in difficulty: A follow-up study.' *Amer. J. Psychiat.* **117**: 727–31.

458 WEDGE, B. M. (ed.) 1958. *Psychosocial Problems of College Men.* Div. of Student Mental Hygiene, Yale Univ.; New Haven, Conn.

459 INT. ASS. UNIVERSITIES, 1958. *Student Mental Health* (Papers Int. Ass. Universities, No. 3). Paris.

INDUSTRIAL MENTAL HEALTH

460 KOEKEBAKKER, J. 1955. 'Mental Health and Group Tensions.' *Bull. World Hlth Org.* **13**: 543–50.

461 LING, T. M. (ed.) 1954. *Mental Health and Human Relations in Industry.* London.

462 LING, T. M. 1955. 'La santé mentale dans l'industrie.' *Bull. World Hlth Org.* **13**: 551–9.

463 MINDUS, E. 1955. 'Outlines of a concept of industrial psychiatry.' *Bull. World Hlth Org.* **13**: 561–74.

464 VEIL, C. 1957. 'Aspects médico-psychologiques de l'industrialisation moderne.' *Rev. int. Travail,* **75**. (English transl.: 'Medical and psychological aspects of modern industry.' *Int. Labour Rev.* **75**.)

465 VEIL, C. 1961. 'Hygiène mentale du travailleur.' In *Traité de psychiatrie: Encyclopédie médico-chirurgicale.* Paris. Tome 3, art. 37960 A50.

466 UNITED KINGDOM. 1958. *Final Report of the Joint Committee on Human Relations in Industry 1954–57; and Report of the Joint Committee on Individual Efficiency in Industry 1953–57.* Dept. Sci. Indust. Res. & Med. Res. Council, London.

467 WFMH. 1948. *Third International Congress on Mental Health, London 1948.* Vol. 4: *Mental Hygiene.* London. Pp. 175–209 (Mental Health in Industry and Industrial Relations).

468 WHO. 1953. Joint ILO/WHO Committee on Occupational Health: 2nd Report. *World Hlth Org. tech. Rep. Ser.* 66. Geneva.

469 WHO. 1957. Joint ILO/WHO Committee on Occupational Health: 3rd Report. *World Hlth Org. tech. Rep. Ser.* 135. Geneva.

470 WHO. 1958. *Human Relations and Mental Health in Industrial Units.* WHO Regional Office for Europe, Copenhagen.

471 WHO. 1959. Mental Health Problems of Automation: Report of a Study Group. *World Hlth Org. tech. Rep. Ser.* 183. Geneva.

PREVENTION OF CRIME AND DELINQUENCY

472 GLUECK, S. & GLUECK, E. T. 1950. *Unraveling Juvenile Delinquency.* New York.

473 GLUECK, S. & GLUECK, E. T. 1959. *Predicting Delinquency and Crime.* Cambridge, Mass.

474 GUTTMACHER, M. S. 1949. 'Medical aspects of the causes and prevention of crime and the treatment of offenders.' *Bull. World Hlth Org.* **2**: 279–88.

475 GUTTMACHER, M. S. 1950. 'Psychiatric examination of offenders.' *Bull. World Hlth Org.* **2**: 743–9.

476 LECONTE, M. 1960. 'De la nécessité de tirer quelques enseignements de l'actualité de la criminalité psychiatrique révélée par la presse.' *Ann. Méd. lég.* **40**: 246–63.

477 LOPEZ-REY, M. 1958. 'Mental health and the work of the United Nations in the field of the prevention of crime and the treatment of offenders.' In *Growing Up in a Changing World.* WFMH, London. Pp. 93–100.

478 ENGLAND & WALES. 1959. *Penal Practice in a Changing Society: Aspects of Future Development (England and Wales).* Home Office, London.

479 ENGLAND & WALES. 1960. *Criminal Law Revision Committee: 2nd Report (Suicide).* Home Office, London.

480 UN DEPT. OF SOCIAL AFFAIRS. 1953. *Int. Rev. crim. Policy.* Special issue on Medical, Psychological, and Social Examination of Offenders.

481 UN DEPT. OF SOCIAL AFFAIRS. 1959. European Consultative Group on the Prevention of Crime and Treatment of Offenders (4th Session, Geneva, 1958). *Int. Rev. crim. Policy* **14**: 59–69.

482 UNESCO. 1957. *The University Teaching of Social Sciences: Criminology.* Paris.

Social and Cross-cultural Aspects
of Mental Health Action

HEALTH AND HUMAN WELFARE

483 BURGESS, A. & DEAN, R. F. A. (eds.) 1962. *Malnutrition and Food Habits* (Report of an International and Interprofessional Conference, Cuernavaca, Mexico, 1960). London.

484 FELIX, R. H. *et al.* 1961. *Mental Health and Social Welfare.* New York.

485 MEERLOO, J. A. M. 1952. 'Contribution of the psychiatrist to the management of crisis situations.' *Amer. J. Psychiat.* 109: 352–5.

486 OPLER, M. K. (ed.) 1959. *Culture and Mental Health: Cross-cultural Studies.* New York.

487 PETRULLO, L. & BASS, B. M. (eds.) 1961. *Leadership and Interpersonal Behavior.* New York.

488 RUBIN, V. (ed.) 1960. *Culture, Society and Health.* New York.

489 WELFORD, A. T. *et al.* (eds.) 1962. *Society: Problems and Methods of Study.* London.

490 JOSIAH MACY, JR FOUNDATION. 1950. *Health and Human Relations in Germany.* New York.

491 JOSIAH MACY, JR FOUNDATION. 1951. *Health and Human Relations in Germany.* New York.

492 *Research into Factors Influencing Human Relations: Report of the International Conference (Nijmegen).* Hilversum, 1956.

493 WFMH. 1959. *Africa: Social Change and Mental Health – Report of a Panel Discussion.* . . . (New York, 23 March 1959). London.

CULTURAL STUDIES

494 BIESHEUVEL, S. 1960. 'Select bibliography on the aptitude of the African south of the Sahara, 1917–1958.' In *Mental*

Disorders and Mental Health in Africa South of the Sahara,
CCTA/CSA Publ. No. 35. London. Pp. 263–9.

495 CAROTHERS, J. C. 1953. *The African Mind in Health and Disease: A Study in Ethnopsychiatry* (World Hlth Org. Monogr. Ser. 17). Geneva.

496 DUBOIS, J. A. 1906. *Hindu Manners, Customs and Ceremonies* (transl. from the French MS (1806) and ed. H. K. Beauchamp). (3rd ed.) Oxford. Pp. 160, 522–41.

497 GEBER, M. & DEAN, R. F. A. 1958. 'Psychomotor development in African children: The effects of social class and the need for improved tests.' *Bull. World Hlth Org.* 18: 471–6.

498 HOFFET, F. 1951. *Psychanalyse de l'Alsace.* Paris.

499 HSU, F. L. K. (ed.) 1961. *Psychological Anthropology: Approaches to Culture and Personality.* Homewood, Illinois.

500 HUGHES, C. C. 1960. *An Eskimo Village in the Modern World.* Ithaca, N.Y.

501 KAPLAN, B. (ed.) 1961. *Studying Personality Cross-culturally.* New York.

502 LA BARRE, W. 1962. *They shall take up Serpents: Psychology of the Southern Snake-handling Cult.* Minneapolis. P. 160.

503 LIPSET, S. M. & LOWENTHAL, L. (eds.) 1961. *Culture and Social Character: The Work of David Riesman Reviewed.* New York.

504 MEAD, M. (ed.) 1953. *Cultural Patterns and Technical Change.* UNESCO, Paris.

505 MEAD, M. 1956. *New Lives for Old: Cultural Transformation – Manus, 1928–1953.* London.

506 MEAD, M. 1959. *An Anthropologist at Work: Writings of Ruth Benedict.* Boston.

507 MEAD, M. & WOLFENSTEIN, M. (eds.) 1955 & 1962. *Childhood in Contemporary Cultures.* Chicago.

508 MEADE, J. E. *et al.* 1961. *The Economic and Social Structure of Mauritius.* London.

509 OPLER, M. K. 1956. 'Ethnic differences in behaviour and psychopathology: Italian and Irish.' *Int. J. soc. Psychiat.* 2: 11–22.

510 SODDY, K. (ed.) 1955–56. *Mental Health and Infant Development* (Proc. WFMH Int. Seminar, Chichester, 1952). Vol. 1: *Papers and Discussions*; Vol. 2: *Case Histories*. 2 vols. London & New York.

511 WAGLEY, C. (ed.) 1952. *Race and Class in Rural Brazil.* UNESCO, Paris.

512 CCTA/CSA. 1960. *CSA Meeting of Specialists on the Basic Psychology of African and Madagascan Populations* (Tananarive, 1959). Publ. No. 51. London.

SOME SOCIAL QUESTIONS

I. *Ageing*

513 TIBBITTS, C. (ed.) 1960. *Handbook of Social Gerontology: Social Aspects of Aging.* Chicago.

514 TIBBITTS, C. & DONAHUE, W. (eds.) 1960. *Aging in Today's Society.* New Jersey.

515 TOWNSEND, P. 1959. 'Social surveys of old age in Great Britain 1945–58.' *Bull. World Hlth Org.* **21**: 583–91.

II. *Industrialization and Urbanization*

516 CLAY, H. M. 1960. *The Older Worker and his Job* (Problems of Progress in Industry, No. 7). London.

517 CROOME, H. 1960. *Human Problems of Innovation* (Problems of Progress in Industry, No. 5). London.

518 FRIEDMAN, G. 1955. *Industrial Society: The Emergence of the Human Problems of Automation.* Glencoe, Ill.

519 RODGER, A. 1959. 'Ten years of ergonomics.' *Nature, Lond.*, **184**: 20–2.

520 SCOTT, J. F. & LYNTON, R. P. 1952. *The Community Factor in Modern Technology.* UNESCO, Paris.

521 THOMSON, D. C. (ed.) 1957. *Management, Labour and Community*, London.

522 VEIL, C. 1957. 'Phénoménologie du travail.' *Evolut. psychiat.* **4**: 693–721.

523 WELFORD, A. T. 1960. *Ergonomics of Automation* (Problems of Progress in Industry, No. 8). London.

524 CARNEGIE STUDY GROUP. 1958. 'Proceedings of the Carnegie Study Group on the basic principles of automation (Geneva, 1957).' *Int. soc. Sci. Bull.* **10**: 1.

525 ILO. 1961. 'Ergonomics: The scientific approach to making work human.' *Int. Labour Rev.* **83**: 1–35.

526 UNESCO. 1956. *The Social Implications of Industrialization and Urbanization in Africa South of the Sahara.* Paris.

527 UNESCO. 1956. *The Social Implications of Industrialization and Urbanization: Five Studies of Urban Populations of Recent Rural Origin in Cities of Southern Asia.* Calcutta.

528 UNITED KINGDOM. 1956. *Automation: A Report on the Technical Trends and their Impact on Management and Labour.* Dept. Sci. Industr. Res., London.

529 UNITED KINGDOM. 1957. *Men, Steel and Technical Change* (Problems of Progress in Industry, No. 1). London.

530 UNITED KINGDOM. 1960. *Woman, Wife and Worker* (Problems of Progress in Industry, No. 10). London.

531 WFMH. 1957. *Mental Health Aspects of Urbanisation* (Report of discussions conducted in the Economic & Social Council Chamber, United Nations, New York, 1957, by WFMH). London.

532 WHO. 1958. Mental Health Aspects of the Peaceful Uses of Atomic Energy: Report of a Study Group. *World Hlth Org. tech. Rep. Ser.* 151. Geneva.

533 WHO. 1960. 'The psycho-social environment in industry.' *World Hlth Org. Chron.* **14**: 276–9.

III. *International Action*

534 BERGER, G. *et al.* 1959. 'Rapports de l'Occident avec le reste du monde.' *Perspectives*, Paris, No. 3 (avril). (Cf. English review: *World ment. Hlth* 1959, **11**: 190–5.)

535 KISKER, G. W. (ed.) 1951. *World Tensions: The Psychopathology of International Relations.* New York.

536 OPLER, M. E. 1954. *Social Aspects of Technical Assistance in Operation.* UNESCO, Paris.

537 UNESCO. 1953. *Interrelations of Cultures: Their Contribution to International Understanding.* Paris.

538 UNESCO. 1957. *The Nature of Conflict: Studies on the Sociological Aspects of International Tensions.* Paris.

539 WFMH. 1955. *Social Implications of Technical Assistance* (Report of a meeting held at the UN, New York, 1955). London.

IV. *Migration and Social Displacement*

540 BORRIE, W. D. *et al.* 1959. *The Cultural Integration of Immigrants.* UNESCO, Paris.

541 CURLE, A. & TRIST, E. 1947. 'Transitional communities and social reconnection.' *Human Relations* 1: 42–68, 240–288.

542 MURPHY, H. B. M. *et al.* 1955. *Flight and Resettlement.* UNESCO, Paris.

543 ILO. 1959. *International Migration, 1945–1957* (Studies and Reports, No. 54). Geneva.

544 ILO. 1961. 'Some aspects of the international migration of families.' *Int. Labour Rev.* **83**: 65–86.

545 WFMH. 1960. *Uprooting and Resettlement* (11th Ann. Meeting WFMH, Vienna, 1958). London.

V. *Population*

546 LORIMER, F. *et al.* 1954. *Culture and Human Fertility.* UNESCO, Paris.

547 PINCUS, G. 1961. 'Suppression of ovulation with reference to oral contraceptives.' In *Modern Trends in Endocrinology,* 2nd ser., ed. H. Gardiner-Hill. London. Pp. 231–45.

548 TITMUSS, R. M. & ABEL SMITH, B. 1961. *Social Policies and Population Growth in Mauritius.* London.

549 'Mauritius and Malthus.' 1961. *Lancet* 1: 542–3.

550 UNITED KINGDOM. 1960. *Report of the Departmental Committee on Human Artificial Insemination.* Home Office & Scottish Home Dept, London.

SOME SOCIAL DIFFICULTIES

I. *Delinquency*

551 ERIKSON, E. H. 1956. *New Perspectives for Research on Juvenile Delinquency.* Washington, D.C.
552 WILKINS, L. T. 1960. *Delinquent Generations.* London.
553 UN DEPT. OF ECON. SOCIAL AFFAIRS (DIV. OF SOCIAL WELFARE). 1952–58. *Comparative Survey on Juvenile Delinquency.* Pt I: North America (revised ed.); Pt II: Europe (in French*); Pt III: Latin America (revised ed.) (in Spanish**); Pt IV: Asia and the Far East; Pt V: Middle East. New York.
(*English summary in *Int. Rev. crim. Policy*, 1954, No. 5: 19–38.)
(**Cf. also J. A. Smythe, 'Juvenile delinquency in Latin American countries.' *Int. Rev. crim. Policy*, 1954, No. 5: 9–18.)

II. *Pathological Attitudes and Mental Disorder*

554 CARSTAIRS, G. M. 1958. 'Some problems of psychiatry in patients from alien cultures.' *Lancet* 1: 1217–20.
555 EISLER, R. 1951. *Man into Wolf: An Anthropological Interpretation of Sadism, Masochism and Lycanthropy.* London.
556 FIELD, M. J. 1955. 'Witchcraft as a primitive interpretation of mental disorder.' *J. ment. Sci.* 101: 826–33.
(Cf. also *J. ment. Sci.* 108: 1043.)
557 GILLIS, L. 1962. *Human Behaviour in Illness: Psychology and Interpersonal Relationships.* With a contribution by S. Biesheuvel. London.
558 JUNG, C. G. 1959. *Flying Saucers: A Modern Myth of Things seen in the Skies* (transl. R. F. C. Hull). London.

559 MEERLOO, J. A. M. 1957. *Mental Seduction and Menticide: The Psychology of Thought Control and Brainwashing.* London.

560 MEERLOO, J. A. M. 1958. ' "Infection mentale": Communication archaïque et régression insensible – Contribution à l'étude psychosomatique des épidémies mentales.' *Méd. et Hyg.*, *Genève*, **16**: 469 et seq.

561 MEERLOO, J. A. M. 1958. 'The delusion of the flying saucer.' *Amer. Practitioner* **9**: 1631–6.

562 MEERLOO, J. A. M. 1959. 'Rock 'n roll: A modern aspect of St Vitus dance – implications for the theory of mental contagion.' *Amer. Practitioner* **10**: 1029–32.

563 SARGANT, W. 1957. *Battle for the Mind: A Physiology of Conversion and Brain-Washing.* London.

564 STENGEL, E. & COOK, N. G. 1958. *Attempted Suicide: Its Social Significance and Effects* (Maudsley Monogr. No. 4). London.

565 WITTKOWER, E. D. & FRIED, J. 1959. 'A cross-cultural approach to mental health problems.' *Amer. J. Psychiat.* **116**: 423–8.

566 CHURCH [OF ENGLAND] ASSEMBLY BOARD FOR SOCIAL RESPONSIBILITY. 1959. *Ought Suicide to be a Crime? – A Discussion of Suicide, Attempted Suicide and the Law.* London.

567 MILBANK MEMORIAL FUND. 1953. *Interrelations between the Social Environment and Psychiatric Disorders.* New York.

III. *Prejudice and Discrimination*

568 ADORNO, T. W. *et al.* 1950. *The Authoritarian Personality.* New York.

569 ALLPORT, G. W. 1954. *The Nature of Prejudice.* Cambridge, Mass.

570 BIESHEUVEL, S. 1959. *Race, Culture and Personality.* Johannesburg.

571 MYERS, J. K. & ROBERTS, B. 1959. *Family and Class Dynamics*. London.

572 GROUP FOR THE ADVANCEMENT OF PSYCHIATRY (GAP). 1957. *Psychological Aspects of School Desegregation* (Report No. 37). New York.

573 UNESCO. 1956. *The Race Question in Modern Science*. Paris.

IV. *Problems of Sex Behaviour*

574 ALLEN, C. 1958. *Homosexuality: Its Nature, Causation and Treatment*. London. (Cf. especially Pt. III: 'Social Significance'; pp. 54–63.)

575 BAILEY, D. S. (ed.) 1956. *Sexual Offenders and Social Punishment*. Church of England Moral Welfare Council, London.

576 FORD, C. S. & BEACH, F. A. 1951. *Patterns of Sexual Behavior*. New York.

577 WESTWOOD, G. 1960. *A Minority: A Report of the Life of the Male Homosexual in Great Britain*. London.

578 BRITISH MEDICAL ASS. 1955. *Homosexuality and Prostitution*. London.

579 UNITED KINGDOM. 1957. *Report of the Committee on Homosexual Offences and Prostitution*. Home Office, Scottish Home Dept, London.

Professional Training

PSYCHIATRY AND THE MEDICAL UNDERGRADUATE

580 BALINT, M. 1961. 'The pyramid and the psychotherapeutic relationship.' (Re: Training of medical students.) *Lancet* 2: 1051–4.

581 BARTON HALL, S., HEARNSHAW, L. S. & HETHERINGTON, R. R. 1961. 'The teaching of psychology in the medical curriculum.' *J. ment. Sci.* 107: 1003–10.

582 CURRAN, D. 1955. 'The place of psychology and psychiatry in medical education.' *Brit. med. J.* 2: 515–18.

583 HARGREAVES, G. R., BROWN, D. G. & WHYTE, M. B. H. 1962. 'Home visits by medical students: An aspect of psychiatric education.' *Lancet* 2: 141–2.

584 HENDERSON, D. 1955. 'Why psychiatry?' *Brit. med. J.* 2: 519–23.

585 HILL, D. 1960. 'Acceptance of psychiatry by the medical student.' *Brit. med. J.* 1: 917–18.

586 LEVINE, M. & LEDERER, H. D. 1959. 'Teaching of psychiatry in medical schools.' In *American Handbook of Psychiatry*, ed. S. Arieti. New York. Vol. 2: 1923–34.

587 MACCALMAN, D. R. 1953. 'Observations on the teaching of the principles of mental health to medical students' (and Memorandum on undergraduate teaching of psychiatry – from the Roy. Med.-Psychol. Ass.). *Brit. J. med. Psychol.* 26: 140–51.

588 PARKER, S. 1960. 'The attitudes of medical students toward their patients: An exploratory study.' *J. med. Educ.* 35: 849–56.

589 RICKLES, N. K. 1960. 'General medicine before specialization.' *Amer. J. Psychiat.* 116: 663.

590 STEVENSON, I. 1961. *Medical History-taking*. New York.

591 TANNER, J. M. 1958. 'The place of human biology in medical education.' *Lancet* 1: 1185–8.

592 TREDGOLD, R. F. 1962. 'The integration of psychiatric teaching into the curriculum.' *Lancet* 1. 1344–7.

593 AMERICAN PSYCHIATRIC ASS. 1952. *Psychiatry and Medical Education.* Washington, D.C.

594 'Psychological medicine and undergraduate education.' 1958. *Brit. med. J.* 2: 602.

595 WHO. 1961. The Undergraduate Teaching of Psychiatry and Mental Health Promotion: 9th Report of the Expert Committee on Mental Health. *World Hlth Org. tech. Rep. Ser.* 208. Geneva.

596 WHO. 1961. *Teaching of Psychiatry and Mental Health* (World Hlth Org. publ. Hlth Papers 9). Geneva.

PSYCHIATRY AND THE MEDICAL POSTGRADUATE

597 BLEULER, M. *et al.* 1961. *Teaching of Psychiatry and Mental Health* (World Hlth Org. publ. Hlth Papers 9). Geneva.

598 DAVIES, T. T., DAVIES, E. T. L. & O'NEILL, D. 1958. 'Case-work in the teaching of psychiatry.' *Lancet* 2: 34–7.

599 GILDEA, E. F. 1959. 'Teaching of psychiatry to residents.' In *American Handbook of Psychiatry*, ed. S. Arieti. New York. Vol. 2: 1935–47.

600 HOLT, R. R. & LUBORSKY, L. 1958. *Personality Patterns of Psychiatrists: A Study of Methods of Selecting Residents.* New York.

601 LEVY, D. M. 1959. *The Demonstration Clinic for the Psychological Study and Treatment of Mother and Child in Medical Practice.* Springfield, Ill.

602 MEARES, A. 1960. 'Communication with the patient.' *Lancet* 1: 663–7.

603 AMERICAN PSYCHIATRIC ASS. 1953. *The Psychiatrist: His Training and Development.* Washington, D.C.

604 ROYAL MEDICO-PSYCHOL. ASS. 1951. *Memorandum on the Training of the Consultant Child Psychiatrist.* London.

605 ROYAL MEDICO-PSYCHOL. ASS. 1960. *The Recruitment and Training of the Child Psychiatrist.* London.

(Cf. Recruitment and training of child psychiatrists. *Brit. med. J.*, 1960. **2**: 205–6.)

PSYCHIATRY AND THE GENERAL PRACTITIONER

606 BALINT, M. 1954. 'Training general practitioners in psychotherapy.' *Brit. med. J.* **1**: 115–20.

607 CARSTAIRS, G. M., WALTON, H. J. & FAWCETT, P. G. 1962. 'General practitioners and psychological medicine: Their views on a postgraduate course.' *Lancet* **2**: 397.

608 GOSHEN, C. E. 1959. 'A project for the creation of better understanding of psychiatry by the general practitioner.' *Southern med. J.* **52**: 30–4.

OTHER PROFESSIONAL TRAINING IN THE MENTAL HEALTH FIELD

609 AFFLECK, J. W. *et al.* 1960. 'In-service mental-health teaching for health visitors.' *Lancet* **2**: 641–3.

610 CAPLAN, G. 1959. 'An approach to the education of community mental health specialists.' *Ment. Hyg.* **43**: 268–80.

611 FERARD, M. L. & HUNNYBUN, N. K. 1962. *The Caseworker's Use of Relationships*. London.

612 JAMES, E. 1958. 'The education of the scientist.' *Brit. med. J.* **2**: 575–6.

613 WRIGHT, M. S. 1962. *An Interim Report on the Characteristics of Successful and Unsuccessful Student Nurses in Scotland*. Edinburgh.
(*As summarized:* Intelligence and student nurses. *Brit. med. J.*, 1962, **2**: 37–8.)

614 AMERICAN ASS. PSYCHIAT. SOCIAL WORKERS. 1950. *Education for Psychiatric Social Work*. New York.

615 (BRITISH) ASS. PSYCHIAT. SOCIAL WORKERS. 1957. *Essentials of Case Work*. London.

616 ENGLAND & WALES. 1962. *The Training of Staff of Training Centres for the Mentally Subnormal*. Ministry of Health

(Central Health Services Council Standing Mental Health Advisory Committee), London.

617 LEVERHULME STUDY GROUP. 1961. *The Complete Scientist: An Inquiry into the Problem of achieving Breadth in the Education at School and University of Scientists, Engineers and other Technologists* (Report of the Leverhulme Study Group to the Brit. Ass. Advance. Sci.). London.

618 'Papers on the Teaching of Personality Development.' 1958. *Sociol. Rev. Monogr.* No. 1.

619 WFMH. 1956. *Mental Health in Teacher Education.* London.

620 WHO. 1956. Expert Committee on Psychiatric Nursing: 1st Report. *World Hlth Org. tech. Rep. Ser.* 105. Geneva.

AUDIO-VISUAL AIDS

621 PILKINGTON, T. L. 1960. 'The use of film in psychiatry.' *World ment. Hlth* 12: 143–5.

622 RUHE, D. S. *et al.* 1960. 'Television in the teaching of psychiatry: Report of four years' preliminary development.' *J. med. Educ.* 35: 916–26.

623 STAFFORD-CLARK, D. *et al.* 1961. 'Television in medical education.' *Brit. med. J.* 1: 500.

CATALOGUES OF FILMS FOR PSYCHIATRIC, PROFESSIONAL, AND PUBLIC EDUCATION:

624 (*a*) Deutsches Zentralinstitut für Lehrmittel. 1960. *Verzeichnis der wissenschaftlichen Filme.* Berlin (East Germany).

625 (*b*) Institut für den wissenschaftlichen Film. 1960. *Gesamtverzeichnis der wissenschaftlichen Filme.* Göttingen (German Federal Republic).

626 (*c*) La Presse Médicale. 1956–57. *Films médicaux et chirurgicaux français*, ed. P. Détrie. Paris, 1956; Supplément, 1957.

627 (*d*) Scientific Film Ass. 1960. *Films of Psychology and Psychiatry.* London.

628   (*e*) U.S. Information Agency. 1956. *United States Educational, Scientific, and Cultural Motion Pictures and Filmstrips: Science Section.* Washington, D.C.

629   (*f*) WFMH. 1960. *International Catalogue of Mental Health Films,* ed. T. L. Pilkington. (2nd ed.) London.

Public Education in Mental Health

PROGRAMMES AND THEIR EVALUATION

630 MEAD, M. 1959. 'Cultural factors in community-education programs.' In *Community Education Principles and Practices from World-wide Experience* (58th Yearbook of the Nat. Soc. for the Study of Education), ed. N. B. Henry. Chicago.

631 POWELL, E. 1961. Everybody's business: Emerging patterns for mental health services and the public (NAMH London Ann. Conf.). As reported in *Brit. med. J.* 1: 820. (Cf. *Lancet* 1: 608–9.)

632 RIDENOUR, N. 1953. 'Criteria of effectiveness in mental health education.' *Amer. J. Orthopsychiat.* 23: 271–9.

633 PENNSYLVANIA MENTAL HEALTH, INC. 1960. *Mental Health Education: A Critique.* Philadelphia.

634 WHO. 1958. Expert Committee on Training of Health Personnel in Health Education of the Public. *World Hlth Org. tech. Rep. Ser.* 156. Geneva.

635 WHO. 1959. Conference on Mental Hygiene Practice (Helsinki, 1959). Report of Committee C: The Education of the Public in Mental Health Principles. WHO Regional Office for Europe, Copenhagen. (Duplicated document.)

PROGRAMMES FOR PARENTS

636 ISAMBERT, A. 1960. *L'Education des parents.* Paris.

637 ISAMBERT, A. 1960. 'Parent education in France.' *World ment. Hlth* 12: 130–3.

638 LEWIS, R. S., STRAUSS, A. A. & LEHTINEN, L. E. 1960. *The Brain-Injured Child: A Book for Parents and Laymen.* (2nd ed.) London.

639 MACKAY, J. L. 1960. 'Parent education in the United States of America.' *World ment. Hlth* 12: 76–85.

640 STERN, H. H. 1960. *Parent Education: An International Survey.* Univ. of Hull, & UNESCO Inst. for Education. Hull.

641 LOUISIANA ASS. MENTAL HEALTH. 1957. *The New Revised and Extended 'Pierre the Pelican' Series.* 28 issues. New Orleans.

POPULAR CONCEPTS OF MENTAL HEALTH

642 CARSTAIRS, G. M. & WING, J. K. 1958. 'Attitudes of the general public to mental illness.' *Brit. med. J.* 2: 594–7.

643 LEMKAU, P. V. & CROCETTI, G. M. 1962. 'An urban population's opinion and knowledge about mental illness.' *Amer. J. Psychiat.* 118: 692–700.

644 NUNNALLY, J. C., JR. 1961. *Popular Conceptions of Mental Health: Their Development and Change.* New York.

645 PAUL, B. D. (ed.) 1955. *Health, Culture and Community: Case Studies of Public Reactions to Health Programs.* New York.

USE OF THE MASS MEDIA

646 ESSEX-LOPRESTI, M. 1961. 'National television programmes.' *Med. biol. Illustr.* 11: 68.

647 JACOBY, A. 1960. 'On using mental health films.' In *International Catalogue of Mental Health Films.* (2nd ed.) WFMH, London. Pp. 6–7.

648 AMERICAN PSYCHIATRIC ASS. 1956. *Psychiatry, the Press and the Public: Problems in Communication.* Washington, D.C.

649 WHO. 1959. *World Health* 12, No. 3 (May–June 1959). Special issue: Mental Health.

650 WHO. 1961. *World Health* 14, No. 4 (July–Aug. 1961). To counter mental illness: Science. A special issue to mark the conclusion of the Mental Health Year (1960–61).

Additional References

651 KAY, D. & ROTH, M. 1961. 'Physical disability and emotional factors in the mental disorders.' Paper read at the IIIrd World Congress of Psychiatry, Montreal, June 1961.

652 SELLIN, T. 1938. 'Culture conflict and crime.' *Soc. Sci. Res. Bull.* **41**; *Am. J. Sociol.* **44**: 97–103.

653 BOWLBY, J. 1960. 'Grief and mourning in infancy and early childhood.' *Psycho-Anal. Study Child* **15**: 9–52.

654 BOWLBY, J. 1961. 'Processes of mourning.' *Int. J. Psycho-Anal.* **42**: 317–40.

655 BOWLBY, J. 1961. 'Childhood mourning and its implications for psychiatry.' *Am. J. Psychiat.* **118**: 481.

656 BUCKLE, D. F. 1962. 'Quelques aspects de l'évolution de la pratique psychiatrique en Europe.' *L'information psychiatrique* **5**: No. 5.
    (in English: 'Some developments of psychiatric practice in Europe.' 1962. *Aust. Psychiat. Bull.* **3**: Nos. 3 & 4.
    in Czech: 'K Vyvoji psychiatrické praxe v Evrope.' 1963. *Cs. Psychiat.* **59**.
    in Greek: 'Exelixis tinés ton efarmogon tis psykiatrikis is tin Evropin.' *Arch. med. Sci.*, Athens, 1962, No. 2.)

657 ZIER, A. & DOSHAY, L. J. 1957. 'Procyclidine hydrochloride ("Kemadrin") treatment of parkinsonism.' *Neurology* **7**: 485–9.

658 SCHWAB, R. S. 1959. 'Problems in the treatment of Parkinson's disease in elderly patients.' *Geriatrics* **14**: 545–58.

659 LINDSAY, T. F. 1961. 'When scientists stop being human.' *Daily Telegraph*, London, 19 January.

660 PENROSE, L. S. 1959. 'The somatic chromosomes in mongolism.' *Lancet* **1**: 710.

661 KORZYBSKI. 1927. *Science and Sanity.*

662 KORZYBSKI. 1931. *Un système non-aristotélien et sa nécessité pour la rigeur en mathématique et en physique.* Communication to the Congress of the American Mathematical Society, New Orleans.

663 MOUNIER, E. 1949. *Le personnalisme.* Paris. Pp. 8–10. (English transl. *Personalism.* London, 1952.)

664 JAQUES, E. 1951. *The Changing Culture of a Factory.* London.

665 PASAMANICK, B. & LILIENFELD, A. M. 1955. 'The association of maternal and foetal factors with the development of mental deficiency.' *J.A.M.A.* **159**: 155–60.

666 STAR, SHIRLEY. 1952. *Attitudes to Mental Illness.* Chicago: National Opinion Research Center Study. (Mimeographed.)

667 RIESMAN, D. 1950. *The Lonely Crowd.* New Haven.

668 MAIN, T. F. 1958. 'Some thoughts on group behaviour.' Paper read at the Davidson Clinic Summer School, Edinburgh, 1958. (Unpublished.)

669 SIGERIST, H. E. 1945. *Civilization and Disease.* New York. Pp. 66–71.

670 CURRAN, D. 1952. 'Psychiatry Ltd.' *J. ment. Sci.* **98**: 373–81.

671 TREDGOLD, R. F. & SODDY, K. 1963. *Tredgold's Textbook of Mental Deficiency.* (10th edition.) London. Pp. 98 and 151–229.

672 MIDDENDORF, W. 1960. *New Forms of Juvenile Delinquency: their Origin, Prevention and Treatment* (2nd UN Congress Prev. Crime & Treat. Offenders). UN Dept. Econ. Social Affairs, New York.

673 LEBOVICI, S. 1959. 'La prévention en santé mentale chez l'enfant.' Réflexions à propos du Seminar de Copenhague sous les auspices de l'Organisation mondiale de la Santé, 1958. *Psychiatrie de l'Enfant* **2**: 197–226.

674 ENGEL, G. L. 1961. 'Is grief a disease?' *Psychosomat. Med.* **23**: 18–22.

675 SPITZ, R. 1945. *The Psychoanalytic Study of the Child* **1**: 53. ibid. 1946, **2**: 113.

Supplementary Titles

ABRAMS, A., TOMAN, J. E. P. & GARNER, H. H. 1963. *Unfinished Tasks in the Behavioral Sciences*. London.

ALLINSMITH, W. & GOETHALS, G. W. 1962. *The Role of Schools in Mental Health*. New York.

APLEY, J. & MACKEITH, R. 1962. *The Child and his Symptoms*. Oxford.

ATKIN, I. 1962. *Aspects of Psychotherapy*. Edinburgh.

BARTON, WALTER. 1962. *Administration in Psychiatry*. Springfield, Illinois.

BOCKHOVEN, J. S. 1963. *Moral Treatment in American Psychiatry*. New York.

BOSCH, GERHARD. 1962. *Der Frühkindliche Autismus*. Berlin, Göttingen, Heidelberg.

CLARK, D. H. 1964. *Administrative Therapy*. London.

COHEN, JOHN. (ed.) 1964. *Readings in Psychology*. London.

CURRAN, D. & PARTRIDGE, M. 1963. *Psychological Medicine*. Edinburgh.

DAVIES, E. B. (ed.) 1964. *Depression* (Proceedings of a symposium by the Cambridge Postgraduate Medical School). London.

DUHL, L. J. (ed.) 1963. *The Urban Condition. People and Policy in the Metropolis*. New York.

EPSTEIN, C. 1962. *Intergroup Relations for Police Officers*. London.

FISH, F. J. 1963. *Clinical Psychiatry for the Layman*. Bristol.

FISH, F. J. 1964. *An Outline of Psychiatry for Students and Practitioners*. Bristol.

FREEMAN, H. E. & SIMMONS, O. G. 1963. *The Mental Patient comes Home*. New York.

GETZELS, J. W. & JACKSON, P. W. 1962. *Creativity and Intelligence: Explorations with Gifted Students*. New York.

GIBSON, J. 1962. *Psychiatry for Nurses*. Oxford.

SUPPLEMENTARY TITLES

GIBSON, J. 1963. *A Guide to Psychiatry*. Oxford.

GILBERT, J. B. 1962. *Disease and Destiny*. London.

GOLDFARB, W. 1961. *Childhood Schizophrenia*. Cambridge, Mass.

HALLAS, C. H. 1962. *Nursing the Mentally Subnormal*. Bristol.

HEATON-WARD, W. A. 1963. *Mental Subnormality*. (2nd ed.) Bristol.

HOLMES, D. J. 1963. *The Adolescent in Psychotherapy*. London.

HOWELLS, J. G. 1963. *Family Psychiatry*. Edinburgh.

ILLINGWORTH, R. S. 1963. *The Normal School Child: His Problems, Physical and Emotional*. London.

JOHN, A. L. 1961. *A Study of the Psychiatric Nurse*. Edinburgh.

JOHNSTON, N., SAVITZ, L. & WOLFGANG, M. E. (eds.) 1962. *The Sociology of Punishment and Correction: A Book of Readings*. New York.

JONES, M. 1962. *Social Psychiatry: in the Community, in Hospitals and in Prisons*. Springfield, Illinois.

KAPLAN, M. 1960. *Leisure in America: a social inquiry*. New York.

KELLNER, R. 1963. *Family Ill Health*. London.

KRAKOWSKI, A. J. & SANTORA, D. A. 1962. *Child Psychiatry and the General Practitioner*. Illinois.

KRAMER, B. M. 1962. *Day Hospital*. New York.

LEIGHTON, A. H. *et al.* 1963. *Psychiatric Disorder among the Yoruba*. New York.

LIN, TSUNG-YI & STANDLEY, C. C. 1962. *The Scope of Epidemiology in Psychiatry* (World Hlth Org. publ. Hlth Papers 16). Geneva.

MACKENZIE, M. 1963. *Psychological Depression: A Common Disorder of Personality*. London.

MADDISON, D. C. 1963. *Psychiatric Nursing*. Edinburgh.

MARKS, P. A. & SEEMAN, W. 1963. *The Actuarial Description of Abnormal Personality*. London.

MCGHIE, A. 1963. *Psychology as applied to Nursing*. Edinburgh.

MOWBRAY, R. M. & RODGER, T. F. 1963. *Psychology in relation to Medicine*. Edinburgh.

OLMSTEAD, C. 1962. *Heads I win, Tails you lose*. New York.

PRONKO, N. H. 1963. *Textbook of Abnormal Psychology.* London.

PUGH, T. F. 1962. *Epidemiologic Findings in United States Mental Hospital Data.* London.

RICHTER, D., TANNER, J. M., TAYLOR, LORD & ZANGWILL, O. L. (eds.) 1962. *Aspects of Psychiatric Research.* London.

RIDENOUR, NINA. 1961. *Mental Health in the United States.* Harvard.

RODGER, T. F., INGRAM, I. M. & MOWBRAY, R. M. 1962. *Lecture Notes on Psychological Medicine.* Edinburgh.

SARGANT, W. & SLATER, E. 1963. *An Introduction to Physical Methods of Treatment in Psychiatry.* Edinburgh.

SARASON, S., DAVIDSON, K. & BLATT, B. 1962. *The Preparation of Teachers.* New York.

SCHIMEL, J. L. 1961. *How to be an Adolescent – and Survive.* New York.

SIM, M. 1963. *Guide to Psychiatry.* Edinburgh.

STAFFORD-CLARK, D. 1964. *Psychiatry for Students.* London.

STEINFELD, J. I. 1963. *A New Approach to Schizophrenia.* London.

TAYLOR, LORD & CHAVE, S. 1964. *Mental Health and Environment.* London.

THOMPSON, G. G. 1962. *Child Psychology.* London.

VALENTINE, M. *An Introduction to Psychiatry.* Edinburgh.

WAHL, C. W. 1963. *Psychosomatic Medicine.* London.

WEINBERG, A. A. 1961. *Migration and Belonging. A Study of Mental Health and Personal Adjustment in Israel.* The Hague.

WELFORD, A. T., ARGYLE, M., GLASS, D. V. & MORRIS, J. N. (eds.) 1962. *Society: Problems and Methods of Study.* New York.

WENAR, C., HANDLON, M. W. & GARNER, A. M. 1962. *Psychosomatic and Emotional Disturbances: A Study of Mother-Child-Relationships* (A Psychosomatic Medicine Monograph). New York.

WOLFGANG, M. E., SAVITZ, L. & JOHNSTON, N. (eds.) 1962. *The Sociology of Crime and Delinquency: a Book of Readings.* New York.

ZILBOORG, G. 1962. *Psychoanalysis and Religion.* New York.

VAN ZONNEVELD, R. J. 1961. *The Health of the Aged.* Edinburgh.

ASSOCIATION OF THE BAR OF THE CITY OF NEW YORK WITH CORNELL UNIVERSITY LAW SCHOOL. 1962. *Mental Illness and Due Process.* New York.

GROUP FOR THE ADVANCEMENT OF PSYCHIATRY (GAP), COMMITTEE ON HOSPITALS. 1963. *Public Relations: A Responsibility of the Mental Hospital Administration.* New York.

Proceedings of the Third World Congress of Psychiatry, Montreal. 1961. Vols I & II. Toronto and Montreal.

ROYAL MEDICO-PSYCHOL. ASS. 1963. *Hallucinogenic Drugs and their Psychotherapeutic Use* (Proceedings of a Meeting of the Association, 1961). London.

SOCIETY FOR PSYCHOSOMATIC RESEARCH. *The Nature of Stress Disorder* (Report of 1958 conference). London.

Index

action research, 211
admission to mental hospitals, *see* mental hospitals
adolescents
  mental health problems of, 131
  mentally defective, training schemes for, 131
  raising the status of, 135
adoption of children, 176, 177
advisory role of voluntary organizations, 221
advisory services, community network of, 121
aetiology, 44
  clinical symptoms and, 40
  of mental disorders, research on, 204–6
  of schizophrenia, research on, 205
aftercare, 96
  of discharged patients, 105, 112
  lack of continuity in, 98
alcohol, physiological intolerance by drugs, 137
Alcoholics Anonymous, 107, 137
alcoholism, 136, 180
  emergency services for, 122
ambulatory mental health services, 107
antabuse, 137
anxiety, optimal level of, 159
ataractic drugs, 84
atmosphere in mental hospitals, 74

babies, handicapped, saving lives of, 180
barbiturates, use of, 89
beds
  in mental hospitals, *see* mental hospitals
  in psychiatric wards in general hospitals, statistics, 113–14
Bio-Sciences Information Exchange, 221
bromides, use of, 89

case-finding
  education of public, 207
  through education system, 179
  training of personnel, 207
central mental health agency, 4
change as cause of social tension, 149

changing conditions of society, studies of, 227
changing environmental factors, 40
child behaviour, research in, 208–10
child guidance, 124, 125
  follow-up studies, 178
child guidance clinics, 126
  slow growth of, 177
child mental health, work in, 18
child psychiatry, 124
childhood schizophrenia, diagnosis of, 45
children
  adoption of, 176, 177
  age at which subject to criminal proceedings, 183
  diagnostic approach, need for reappraisal of, 48
  difficulties in relationship with other peoples', 191
  disaster, effects on, 184
  disturbed, 127
  family structure, effects on, 187–92
  in hospital, 127
    admittance of mother, 128
    unrestricted visiting, 128
  intelligence tests, 206
  maladjusted, provision for, 126
  maternal deprivation in, 127
  mental health problems, 124–30
  mentally handicapped, formation of parent associations, 130
  psychological tests on, 43
  psychotic
    and relationship with mother, 49
    shortage of accommodation for, 127
    and psychotic parent, 94
  retarded, educational facilities for, 130
  social services for, 125
  see also mother–child relationship
chronic mental patients
  care of, 67
  discharge of, 93
  employment of, 110, 111
  rehabilitation centres for, 68
chronicity in long-stay patients, reduction of, 77
church in mental health problems, function of, 9

299

maladjusted children, provisions for, 126
marriage guidance, 183
mass migration of rural populations, effects of, 185
maternal deprivation, 127, 176
maternal function in mental health, 182
medical training, 160
meningitis, 176
mental defectives, in foster homes, 123, 131
rehabilitation of, 132
useful employment in wartime, 132
mental deficiency, 129
metabolic origins of, research into, 197, 198
mental disorder
clinical picture of, and changing environmental factors, 40
diagnosis of, in different cultures, 41
epidemiological method, application to, 158
primary prevention, 173, 174–7
quarternary prevention, 185
recognition of, 37–56
research in pathology of, 204–6
research on aetiology of, 204–6
secondary prevention, 173, 177–80
tertiary prevention, 173, 180–5
mental health
check-ups, 55
and community planning, 162
human relations aspects in, 164
implications in other fields, 160
in industry, 184, 229
maternal function in, 182
planning in United Kingdom, 12
planning trends in United States, 7
prophylaxis in, 173–92
research in, see research
social issues affecting, 202
tension and, interdependence, 36
Mental Health Act (1959), 13, 15, 60, 99, 130, 153
mental health action in the community, 153–72
mental health agencies, 158
mental health associations, national, organization, 26
mental health centres, 104
area coverage, 106
functions of, 105
mental health observation, scientific techniques for, 196
mental health organizations
evaluation of, 155–7
structural problems, 28

mental health problems
of adolescents, 131
of children, 124–30
in society, 119–37
mental health projects, index of, 224
mental health publications in other fields, 161
mental health services
ambulatory, 107
citizen groups, participation in, 158
community, 119
and community services, need for integration, 5
current trends in development, 15
in developing countries, 143
in different cultures, 20–22
district, 107
extramural, 99
mobile, in rural districts, 107
planning, clinical community trends, 3
planning and organizing cross-culturally, 149–52
on regional basis, 6
student, 129
mental health societies, harnessing energy and enthusiasm of members, 35
mental health techniques, international application of, 162
mental hospitals, 57–82
admission, 57
admission of unwilling patients, legal powers to compel, 58
admission rates, 62
increase in, 63, 71
atmosphere in, 74
bed provision, planning, 64
beds occupied, decline in, 63
beds, reduction in numbers, 99
beds, shortage of, 3
community and, relationships between, 97
community attitudes to, 92
discharge from, see discharge
discharge rates, 72
duration of stay, 63
flexibility of, 68
and general hospitals, intercommunication, 6
old-style, conditions in, 66
permissiveness in, 80
population, 62
practice, effects of current trends, 91–101
psycho-analysis in, role of, 83
readmission rates, increase in, 69
reputation in the community, 91